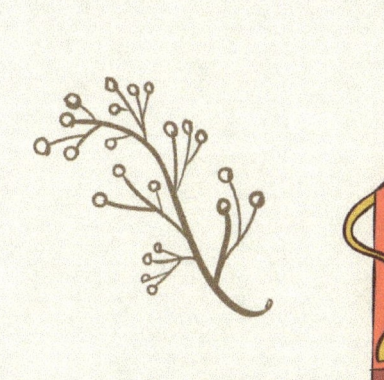
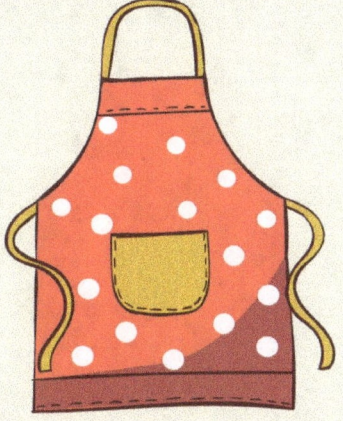

Back to the Kitchen
and enjoying it!

by Ruth Adler Torres

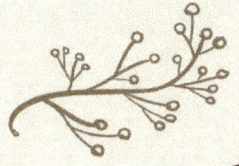
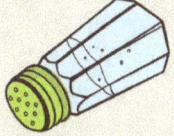
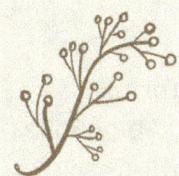
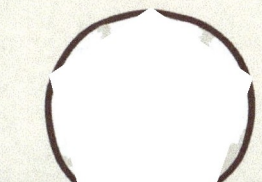

Copyright © 2023 by Dennis Torres

ALL RIGHTS RESERVED
This book contains material protected under International and Federal Copyright Laws and Treaties. Any unauthorized reprint or use of this material is prohibited. No part of this book may be reproduced or transmitted in any form or by any means, electronic or mechanical, including photocopying, recording or by any information storage and retrieval system without express written permission from the author/publisher.

Publisher, Dennis Torres
Hardback ISBN: 978-0-9980824-9-3
Paperback ISBN: 978-0-9980824-6-2

Contact Dennis Torres: DennisTorresMalibu@gmail.com

Foreward by Dennis Torres

The recipes contained in this book were created by my mother Ruth Adler Torres while my sister and I were growing up in the ethnically diverse, working-class town of Perth Amboy, New Jersey. During that time, I was often by my mother's side in the kitchen where I would sample the food coming right out of the oven or from the stove top.

These recipes are a product of her love for cooking and family, but additionally tell a story of the post-World War II cultural revolution, which was as profound, if not more so, than that of the post-Vietnam War era. When the War ended in victory and the USA emerged as a superpower, tens of thousands of young men returned home to their wives and girlfriends amid celebration and optimism for the future. What followed was an unprecedented period of American growth and prosperity. Marriage rates soared, as did the birth rate. The population grew at twice the rate it had grown in the previous decade, giving rise to the popular term "baby boom." Home ownership, particularly in the newly created suburbs, also grew exponentially.

It was a time when women who had traditionally stayed home to care for the children entered the workforce. With this dual income and the introduction of credit cards, Americans had more money to spend than ever before, and the average income of most individuals nearly doubled. At the same time, the GDP grew one hundred fifty percent. As a result, the period became known as America's Golden Era.

Culturally it was also an era of conformity. Men and women accepted their gender roles. Girls didn't wear pants and jeans were forbidden in schools and colleges. Families respected their political leaders, clergy, and the police. Children respected their parents and teachers. Families felt safe in their neighborhoods and children played outside unsupervised for hours. More profoundly it was a time when families sat down and ate together undistracted by any media and engaged in conversation about their lives.

Because women were employed outside the home and responsible for the household, the foods they prepared changed, and recipes changed too. Quick well balance dinners like beef stroganoff, meat loaf, Salisbury steak were popular as were Casseroles like tuna noodle that could be quickly made with inexpensive canned foods; just mix a can of tuna with a can of peas, or corn, a can of cream of mushroom soup, some shredded

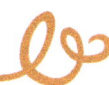

Cheddar cheese, top it off with a can of crispy onions or potato chips and bake. Meat stews, corned beef and cabbage, chicken pot pies, glazed ham creamed onions and peas, cream of celery soup, chicken croquettes, Jell-o salads, mashed potatoes, French fries, and processed foods like the newly introduced Swanson's TV dinners were popular too.

Meals were mostly protein and vegetables. The potions were smaller than those consumed in the decades that followed and people were more physically active so being overweight was rare.

In her Preface my mother references the 1930s because that's the era she grew up in and she had fond memories of her own mother preparing food for the family, but her recipes are decidedly post War 1940s and 1950s. Being the daughter of European Jewish immigrants some of her recipes reflect traditional Ashkenazi foods. And there's even one for Plantains as a salute to her husband's (my father's), Latin heritage.

When she passed away on November 2nd, 1972, my mother left behind her husband Joe, me and my wife Averi, my sister Sharyn and her husband Jerry, and four grandchildren, Mark, Alison, Amy and Jason. Her recipes then became both a medium for our remembrance and a part of her legacy.

She had hoped to get Back To The Kitchen And Enjoying It published to share her joy of cooking and baking, but unfortunately her failing health sidetracked that effort. Years later her eldest granddaughter Alison reproduced the book in a hand typed spiral bound edition as a tribute to her beloved grandmother. This published edition completes my mother's dream. I hope you enjoy the gastronomic and historical journey it offers.

Dennis Torres

Dedicated to my husband Joe,
who has complimented me
and my cooking for thirty-three years.

*In Memory of my Grandmother to preserve
her best recipes for Grandpa, Sharyn,
Dennis, Amy, Jason, Mark and myself, I am
retyping her cookbook for all to have.*

*We can try these recipes, but we know that
Grandma's always tasted better.*

**WE WILL NEVER FORGET YOU -
GRANDMA RUTH A. TORRES**

revised by Alison Rosenberg
(eldest granddaughter)

Preface

The era of nostalgia is upon us. As we look about us we cannot escape some reference to the thirties.

The thirties bring to my mind the closeness of the family structure, mom in the kitchen and the aroma of good cooking.

There was a feeling of belonging and being loved when the family would gather together at the dinner table for a good home cooked meal.

Be that as it may we cannot dwell in the past. We must accept progress and we do so gladly. Who would want to give up our wonderful modern labor saving devices, our super market's freezers bulging with quick frozen vegetables, fruits, pies, cakes and complete meals. The rows upon rows of wonderful convenience foods.

There is a time and place for everything.

There is nothing that takes the place of home cooking, but in this hurried life, that most of us lead, we must at times resort to the easy way out.

With the recipes in this book, I am endeavoring, with the least amount of effort to bring back home cooked food and I hope a little more family togetherness.

Most of the recipes require a short cooking period, many can be prepared in the morning and popped into the oven for a few minutes before serving time.

We can no longer be slaves in our kitchen but we must also not forsake our homes and families.

So back to the kitchen, women. With a little time and love perhaps we can recapture the thirties and have our families together enjoying mom's creative efforts.

Ruth Torres, 1971
(December 12, 1917 - November 2, 1972)

ABBREVIATIONS

t	-	teaspoon
T	-	tablespoon
C	-	cup
oz.	-	ounce or ounces
sq.	-	square
b.p.	-	baking powder
b.s.	-	baking soda
lb.	-	pound
pkg.	-	package

What & Where

PANCAKES & QUICK BREADS 9
APPETIZERS & SALADS 13
MEATS FISH & CHICKEN 23
CASSEROLES & PASTA 35
VEGETABLES & SOUPS 41
SANDWICHES 55
CAKES, PIES & COOKIES 59
FROSTINGS, FILLINGS & SAUCES 77
DESSERTS 83
MISCELLANEOUS 87

Pancakes & Quickbreads

Breakfast should not be overlooked, as it is the most important meal of the day.

The new quick breakfast drinks on the market leave much to be desired when contrasted with eggs, ham, bacon, sausages, cereals, hot and cold etc.

Vary the fruits and juices, the breads, rolls, pancakes, etc.

Variety is still the "spice of life", so spice it with a few changes.

BREAKFAST PANCAKES

- 1 C Bisquick
- 1 egg
- 1 T melted butter
- ¼ t vanilla
- ½ C milk

Mix all ingredients well with whisk or egg beater. Use about 2 T of butter on your griddle and when hot drop pancake batter, about ¼ C for each.

When bubbles form on the surface of pancakes, turn. Makes about 10 small pancakes.

PANCAKE VARIATIONS

Using the basic recipe; add the following:

- **1 C chopped tart apple:** serve with sour cream, sprinkle with sugar & cinnamon
- **1 C blueberries:** serve with blueberry sauce
- **1 C crushed pineapple:** serve with powdered sugar
- **1 banana, sliced:** serve with boysenberry sauce
- **½ C flaked coconut and ½ C chopped pecans:** serve with maple syrup

PINEAPPLE BREAKFAST CAKE

- 2 C Flour
- 2 t baking powder
- ½ t baking soda
- ½ t salt
- ½ C brown sugar
- ½ C pecans, chopped
- 1 egg, beaten
- 1 C sour cream
- 1 8¾ oz. can crushed pineapple, undrained
- ⅓ C oil

Mix all dry ingredients together. Combine egg and cream. Stir in undrained pineapple, oil and nuts.

Bake in 8 or 9 inch greased pan 375 degrees 25-30 minutes. May also be baked in muffin tins (400 degrees for 20 minutes).

CARROT MUFFINS

- 2 C flour
- ¼ c sugar
- 1 T baking powder
- 1 t salt
- 1 C grated raw carrot
- ¾ C milk
- ½ C chopped nuts
- ¼ C oil
- 1 egg, beaten
- 1 t grated orange peel

Stir together flour, sugar, baking powder and salt.

Combine carrot, milk, nuts, oil, egg and orange peel. Add carrot mixture all at once to flour mixture, stirring only until flour is moistened.

Fill greased muffin cups two thirds full; bake at 425 degrees 20 to 25 minutes. Makes 12 muffins.

CORN CHEESE MUFFIN

- 1 C flour
- 1 t salt
- 2 ½ t baking powder
- ¼ C sugar
- 1 C yellow corn meal
- ⅔ C grated American cheese
- 1 C milk
- 1 well beaten egg
- 2 T melted margarine

Mix first six ingredients, add milk, egg and margarine. Mix until moistened. Fill muffin tins two-thirds full. Bake 400 degrees 25 minutes.

ORANGE NUT BREAD

- 2 ¼ C flour
- ¾ C sugar
- ¾ C chopped nuts
- 1 T orange peel
- ¾ C orange juice
- 2 ¼ t baking powder
- ¾ t salt
- ¼ t soda
- 1 beaten egg
- 2 T oil

Mix dry ingredients together, make a well in center and add liquids and nuts. Mix until well blended.

Pour into 9"X 5" loaf pan. Bake 55-60 minutes 350 degrees. Turn out on rack to cool. Wrap in aluminum foil for a day. Slice thin.

MUFFINS

- 1 ½ C flour
- ½ C sugar
- 2 t baking powder
- ½ t salt
- ¼ C soft shortening
- 1 egg
- ½ C milk

Mix together until ingredients are blended. Do not over mix. Fill greased muffin tins 2/3 full. Bake 400 degrees for 20-25 minutes.

VARIATIONS ON MUFFINS

1. Plum muffin: Place 1 canned pitted plum in center of each muffin and top with topping.

2. Blueberry muffin: Add 1 C fresh or well drained frozen blueberries Dust with confectioner's sugar, when cool

3. Date & Nut muffins: Add ¾ C chopped dates and 1/4 C chopped nuts.

4. Apple muffins: Add ½ t cinnamon, ¼ t ground cloves and 1 C grated apple. Top with topping.

TOPPING

- ⅓ C brown sugar
- ⅓ C chopped nuts
- ½ t cinnamon

BANANA NUT BREAD

- 1¾ C flour
- 2 t baking powder
- ¼ t baking soda
- ½ t salt
- ⅓ C shortening
- ⅔ C sugar
- 2 eggs, beaten
- ½ C chopped nuts
- 1 C mashed ripe bananas

Cream shortening and sugar, add eggs and beat until light and fluffy. Beat in dry ingredients, which have been mixed together; alternately with bananas. Bake in greased 9"X 5" loaf pan for about 1 hour. Cool for a few minutes before removing from pan.

Appetizers & Salads

Appetizers are served to whet your appetite, but really, unless you have just one (and who can?) you will have lost your appetite before the meal starts.

Salads come in all shapes, sizes and combinations. They can be used as the first course or the meal itself; either time as an accompaniment to the meal.

I did not think it necessary to include the ever popular tossed salad, but I would like to mention to be sure the greens are well washed, dried, cold and crisp.

Vary the dressings, add croutons, garlic, cheese or plain, for that added crunch.

CHICKEN LIVER APPETIZER

- 7 chicken livers, cut in halves or thirds
- ⅓ C corn meal
- ¼ C flour
- 1 egg, beaten
- 2 T milk
- salt, pepper and garlic powder

Mix egg and milk. Mix dry ingredients, add seasoning. Dip livers in dry ingredients, then egg mix, then dry mix. Fry in deep fat for about 2 minutes. Drain.

FRIED CHICKEN HORS D'OEUVRES

- 3 whole chicken breasts
- 1 egg, beaten
- ½ C flour
- ½ C water
- ¾ t salt
- 1½ C oil

Skin and cut chicken into 1 inch chunks. Mix egg and water, add flour and salt and mix into a batter. Dip chicken in batter and fry in oil 3-5 minutes. Drain and serve with following dipping sauce. Serves about 6.

DIPPING SAUCE

- ⅓ C ketchup
- ¼ t dry mustard
- ½ T brown sugar
- 1 T vinegar
- 3 T margarine

Mix all ingredients together, cook and stir 5 minutes. Pour in bowl and let each person dip the chicken in sauce. Cold plum sauce may also be used for dipping.

CHOPPED LIVER

- 1 lb. beef liver
- 2 eggs, hard cooked
- 1 large onion, chopped
- salt and pepper
- 4 T chicken fat mayonnaise or oil

Cut liver in chunks and fry with onions in 2 T shortening. When well done, put through food chopper with eggs.

Use all the drippings from pan. Add the other 2 T shortening, salt and pepper. Mash with fork. Liver should form a soft paste. Add fat if needed.

Serve cold as appetizer.

PARTY NIBBLERS

- 1 stick margarine
- ½ t garlic powder
- salt
- 3 C mixed dry cereals, rice chex, wheat chex, cheerios
- ½C sunflower seeds, shelled
- ½ C red skins salted peanuts
- 1 C pretzel stix

Melt margarine and seasonings, add cereal and nuts. Place in oven on cookie sheet for 35 minutes 250 degrees.

Stirring occasionally. Remove from oven and add pretzel sticks. Cool then store in air-tight container.

STUFFED TOMATO, 3 Ways

VERSION 1

- 2 Avocados, mashed
- 4 bacon strips, fried crisp & crumbled
- 3 green onions, chopped
- 4 black olives, chopped
- 2 large solid tomatoes, cut in halves and chopped
- Tomato pulp
- salt and pepper

Mash all ingredients except tomatoes. Pile on scooped out tomato halves.

VERSION 2

- 2 large solid tomatoes
- 1 pint creamed cottage cheese
- ½ cucumber, chopped
- salt and pepper

Mix cheese and cucumber; season. Pile on tomato halves.

VERSION 3

- 4 medium tomatoes, scooped
- 1 medium cucumber, diced
- 4 red radishes, chopped
- 4 green onions, sliced
- 1 cold boiled potato, diced (optional)
- tomato pulp
- 1 C sour cream
- 1/2 C cottage cheese
- salt and pepper

Mix all ingredients except tomatoes; season. Fill each tomato very full.

CUCUMBER SALAD

- 1 lg. cucumber, thinly sliced and peeled
- 1 t salt

Cover and let stand for several hours. Pour off liquid and squeeze as much juice from cucumber as you can; mix in jar and shake well.

CUCUMBER RELISH

- ¼ C vinegar
- 2 T oil
- 2 T sugar
- ¼ t celery or dill seed

Pour over cucumbers and refrigerate for several hours in covered container. Serve as a relish.

COMBINATION SALAD

- 1 medium size can garbanzo beans, drained
- 3 green onions, sliced thin
- ½ green pepper, sliced thin
- 2 tomatoes, cut into quarters
- salt and pepper

Marinate in Italian dressing several hours or overnight. Serve on lettuce as salad. Serves 4.

BEAN SALAD

- 8 oz. can cut string beans
- 8 oz. can red kidney beans
- 8 oz. can cut wax beans
- 8 oz. can garbanzos

Drain and rinse each can of vegetables. Mix the beans together in a bowl add 1 thinly sliced onion, separate the slices.

DRESSING

- ½ C vinegar
- 2 T sugar
- ¼ C oil

Shake well. Pour over beans and onions, add salt and pepper and 1/2 t celery seed. Put into a jar or plastic container and refrigerate over night. Turn jar up side down several times during refrigeration. Serve cold.

STUFFED AVOCADO SALADS, 3 Ways

VERSION 1

- 2 avocados, peeled, cut in halves and sprinkled with lemon juice
- 1 can white tuna fish, drained and chopped
- 1 hard cooked egg, chopped
- ½ C celery, chopped
- 2 green onions, chopped
- 4 green or black olives, chopped

Mix all ingredients, except avocado, together. Add enough mayonnaise to hold together. Fill avocado halves.

VERSION 2

- 2 avocados, cut in halves and sprinkled with lemon juice
- 1 lb. can small red kidney beans, drained
- 1 C cooked elbow macaroni
- ½ C mayonnaise
- ½ C grated processed or Jack cheese
- salt and pepper
- dash of chili powder
- garlic powder

Mix together and add seasoning. Fill avocados.

VERSION 3

- 2 avocados, cut in halves
- 1 pint cottage cheese
- 8 oz. can fruit cocktail, drained
- ½ C sour cream
- 1 T sugar
- 4 maraschino cherries

Mix ingredients together. Fill avocados and top with cherries

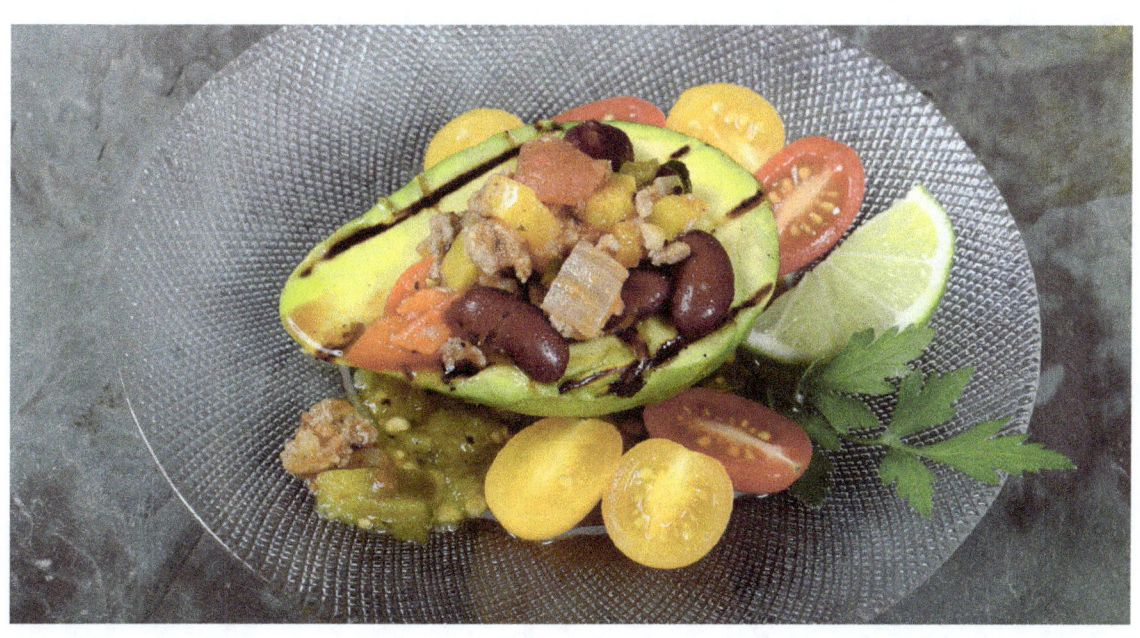

COLE SLAW, Version 1

- 1 small cabbage, shredded
- 2 carrots, grated
- ½ green pepper, chopped

Mix together and add dressing below.

DRESSING

- ½ C mayonnaise plus 2 T vinegar or lemon juice
- 1 T milk
- ½ t salt
- 1 t sugar

Mix well and pour over cole slaw, tossing well to distribute the dressing.

COLE SLAW, Version 2

- 1 small head cabbage, shredded
- 1 medium carrot, grated
- 1/2 green pepper, thinly sliced
- 2-3 green onions, thinly sliced
- 2-3 red radishes, thinly sliced

Mix together and add dressing below.

DRESSING

- ⅔ C vinegar plus 4 T sugar, shake well in jar
- 2 T oil
- 1 t salt

Shake vigorously. Pour over cole slaw, tossing with fork. Place in container with tight cover. Turn up side down a few times, then place in refrigerator for at least 2 hours before serving.

Turn up side down and shake to distribute dressing before serving. Serves 4-6.

HAWAIIAN COLE SLAW

- 1 small head cabbage, shredded
- ½ C chopped walnuts
- 8 oz. can crushed pineapple, drained
- ½ tart apple, chopped (optional)

Mix together and add dressing below.

DRESSING

- ½ C mayonnaise
- 3 T pineapple juice
- ¼ t salt

Place in jar with tight cover. Shake vigorously and pour over slaw. Let stand in refrigerator for at least 2 hours before serving. Serves 4-6.

POTATO SALAD

- 5 large potatoes, cooked and diced
- ¾ C mayonnaise
- 2 hard cooked eggs, chopped
- ½ C celery, sliced
- 1 carrot, grated
- 2 green onions, sliced thin
- salt and pepper
- ¼ t dill weed

Mix all ingredients together, season to taste. Cover and chill before serving. Serves 6.

HOT POTATO SALAD

- 6 slices bacon
- 1 medium onion, chopped
- 2 hard cooked eggs
- 6 cups hot cubed or sliced potatoes
- ⅓ C vinegar
- 2 T sugar

Fry bacon with onions until bacon is crisp. Pour off fat. Crumble bacon and add with onions to potatoes. Mix vinegar and sugar and pour over potatoes. Add salt and pepper to taste. Toss lightly. Garnish with chopped eggs and parsley.

SPINACH SALAD

- 1 bunch spinach leaves, washed drained and stems removed
- 2 hard cooked eggs, chopped
- 6 slices bacon, cooked crisp, drained and crumbled
- Italian dressing or oil and vinegar

Tear spinach into large pieces. Add dressing and toss until well coated. Add egg and bacon and toss again. Sprinkle with grated Parmesan cheese.

MELON RING FRUIT SALAD

- 1 Honeydew or Cantaloupe
- 1 Grapefruit cut into segments
- 1 lg. navel orange, cut into segments
- 1 (8oz.) can pineapple chunks
- About ten maraschino cherries, cut in halves, plus cherry juice

Remove melon rind and seeds. Slice melon into rings. Mix fruits together, adding all the juices including some cherry juice. Let stand for about 30 minutes in refrigerator.

To serve, place on ring or lettuce lined salad plate, fill center with well drained fruit. Top with fruit dressing if desired.

Serve with date and nut bread and butter sandwiches.

FRUIT SOUR CREAM SALAD

- 1 can mandarin oranges
- 1 lb. can fruit cocktail, drained
- 1 9 oz. can crushed pineapple, drained
- 2 C miniature marshmallows
- ½ C coarsely chopped walnuts or pecans
- 1 C sour cream

Combine all ingredients. Cover and chill several hours. Serve on lettuce leaves, sprinkle with coconut before serving. Serves 6-8.

LIME-COTTAGE CHEESE-PINEAPPLE SALAD

- 3 oz. package lime gelatin
- 1 C creamed cottage cheese
- ½ C sour cream
- ½ C crushed pineapple, well drained

Prepare gelatin as directed off package, using the pineapple juice as part of the liquid. Set in refrigerator.

When gelatin is slightly thickened, beat at high speed until fluffy. Add sour cream and blend.

Fold in cheese and pineapple. Pour into 8 inch square pan. When jelled, cut in squares and serve on lettuce.

CRANBERRY NUT SALAD

- 3 oz. package cherry flavored gelatin
- 1-lb. can whole cranberry sauce
- ½ C walnuts, chopped
- ½ t grated orange rind
- ½ t lemon juice

Prepare gelatin as directed on package. Cool for 10 minutes. Add rest of the ingredients. Pour into custard cups.

When jelled, unmold and serve on lettuce.

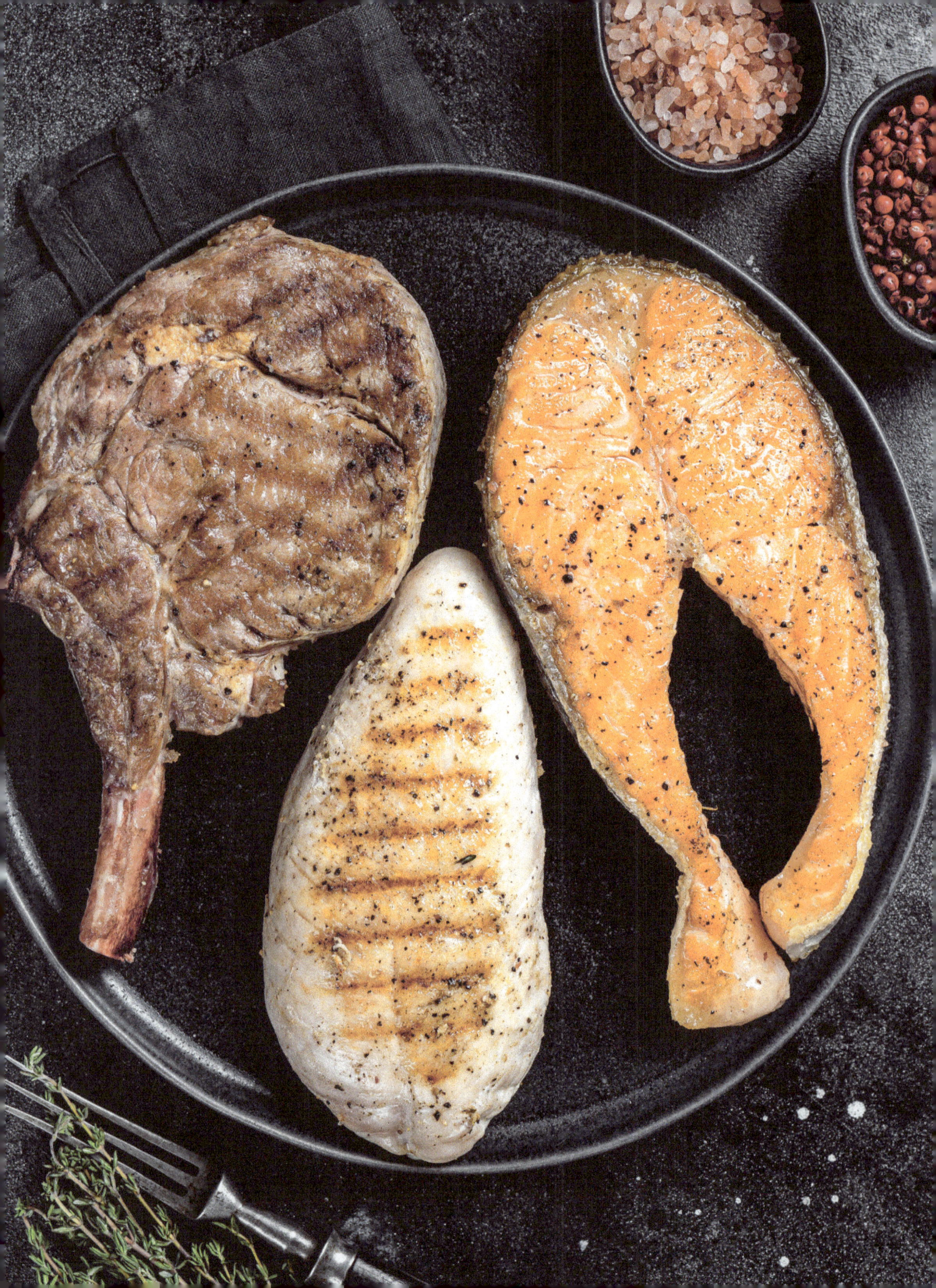

Meats, Fish & Chicken

Prime rib and steaks are always welcome and delicious, but for those of us who budget our food dollar, cooking with cheaper cuts commands a greater challenge.

It is difficult to judge how many portions each recipe serves as appetites vary in each home. Since this book is written for people who can cook, they will be able to judge by the ingredients.

By normal standards, what ever they are, most recipes serve four.

BEEF STEW, Version 1

- 2 lbs. lean beef, cut in cubes
- ¼ C flour
- ¼ t pepper
- 2 t salt
- 1 Bouillon cube
- ¼ t garlic powder
- ½ t paprika
- 2 small onions, sliced
- 2 C boiling water

Place flour, pepper, salt, paprika and garlic powder in plastic bag. Shake meat a few pieces at a time so they become well coated. Brown meat on all sides in oil, then add onions, water and cubes. Bring to boil, then lower flame to simmer. Simmer for 2 hours or until fork tender. Taste for seasoning. Add water or tomato juice if liquid is needed.

Serve with cubed boiled potatoes, sliced carrots and cooked frozen Lima beans.

BEEF STEW. Version 2

- 2 lbs. lean beef, cut in cubes
- ¼ C flour
- pepper, salt, garlic powder
- 1 Bay leaf
- 2 small onions, sliced
- 2 C boiling water
- 1 (8oz) can tomato sauce
- 2 potatoes, diced
- 1 pkg. frozen mixed vegetables

Place flour, salt, pepper, garlic powder in plastic bag. Shake meat a few pieces at a time to coat well.

Brown meat in vegetable shortening or oil until brown on all sides. Add onions, water, bay leaf and tomato sauce; simmer for 1-1/2 hours or until meat is tender.

Taste for seasoning and add potatoes and frozen vegetables. Cook for 15-20 minutes. Serve with broad noodles or plain.

ROAST BRISKET

- 3-4 lbs. brisket
- 1 envelope onion soup mix
- 1 clove garlic (optional)

Rub meat on all sides with garlic. Place on large sheet of aluminum foil. Cover meat with soup mix and fold foil over to cover tightly. Place in 350 degrees oven for 2 hours, then open top of foil and continue roasting for about 35-40 minutes or until meat is tender and browned. Slice and serve.

MEXICAN BEEF STEW

- 2 lbs. lean stew meat
- 1 lg. onion, sliced
- 1 t chili powder
- 1 clove garlic
- Salt and pepper to taste
- 1 can beef broth, plus ½ C water or 1 beef cube in 1-½ C of hot water
- 15 oz. can red kidney beans

Brown meat in oil, add onion and crushed garlic, sprinkle with salt, pepper and chili powder. Add liquid, cover and simmer about 1-1/2 hours until fork tender. Taste to adjust seasonings. Add beans. Serve over rice. Serve with steamed buttered tortillas.

MEAT LOAF

- 2 lbs. ground beef salt and pepper
- 2 eggs
- 2 T chopped onion
- ½ C hot milk
- ½ C flavored bread crumbs
- 2 T dried vegetable flakes
- 8oz. can tomato sauce, plain or with mushrooms

Mix all ingredients together well, except use half of the tomato sauce. Fit into loaf pan or shape into loaf in shallow baking dish. Pour remaining tomato sauce over loaf. Bake about 1 hour 15 minutes 350 degrees.

ROLLED MEAT LOAF

- 2 lbs. ground beef
- 2 eggs
- ½ C bread crumbs
- ½ C hot milk
- 2 T ketchup salt and pepper
- 6 strips of bacon

Mix bread crumbs and hot milk and add to rest of ingredients. Mix well. Pat meat on waxed paper until it is ½ inch thick. Spread with bread stuffing; roll as for jelly roll. Place bacon strips across top. Bake 1½ hours at 350 degrees.

BAR B-Q MEAT BALLS

- 1 ½ lbs. ground beef
- 1 egg
- ½ C bread crumbs
- salt and pepper

Mix and shape into meat balls.

SAUCE

- 1 C ketchup
- ½ C water
- 1 T worchestershire sauce
- 2 T brown sugar
- 2 T vinegar
- ¼ t salt
- ½ large onion, chopped

Mix all ingredients together until well blended. Place meat balls in 2-1/2 qt. casserole dish, pour sauce over them. Bake for 1 hour in 350 degrees covered. Can also be simmered on top of stove for 35 minutes.

Delicious served as Hors d'oeuvres. Pour off sauce and serve hot.

FRUITED POT ROAST

- 3 - 3½ lbs. pot roast
- flour, salt, pepper
- bay leaf
- 2 C water
- ½ C dried prunes
- ½ C dried apricots

Dredge pot roast with flour, salt and pepper. Brown in vegetable shortening until brown on all sides. Add water and bay leaf. Simmer until tender. Remove meat, add fruit and cook for 15 minutes more. Thicken gravy with flour.

To serve, slice meat and pass fruited gravy.

SAVORY POT ROAST

- 3 ½ - 4 lb. chuck roast
- 2 C sliced onions
- ¼ C water
- ¼ C ketchup
- ⅓ C dry red wine
- 1 clove garlic, crushed
- 1 bay leaf
- 2 T flour
- ¼ t marjoram, rosemary & thyme

Dredge meat with flour. Brown in oil. Sprinkle with salt, pepper; add onions. Stir ketchup, wine, garlic and seasonings into water and pour over meat. Cover and simmer about 2 hours. Remove meat, skim off as much fat as you can; add flour to water and stir until smooth. Add to pan drippings and stir until thickened. Slice meat and return to gravy.

STUFFED CABBAGE

- 1 medium head leafy green cabbage
- 1 lb. ground beef
- 1 egg
- salt and pepper
- ¼ C rice (regular)
- 1 lb. 12 oz. can tomatoes, strained
- juice of ½ lemon
- 2½ T sugar
- 1 medium onion, sliced

Cut core from cabbage and put in pot. Cover with water and bring to a boil. Remove from heat and let stand about 10 minutes. Drain and cool, then remove leaves gently, cut off hard edge of each leaf. Mix meat, rice, salt, pepper and egg well. Place about a heaping tablespoonful on each leaf and turn up bottom, then sides, then roll. Place in pan, seam sides down. When all rolls are made, slice onion, add to strained tomato, lemon juice and sugar mixture. Pour over cabbage rolls, cook over low heat for about 1 hour.

Adjust seasoning; it should have a sweet and sour flavor. More lemon juice and sugar may be added.

ORIENTAL STEAK STRIPS

- 1 lb. sirloin steak, cut in narrow strips
- 1 medium onion, sliced thin
- 5 oz. can water chestnuts (drained and sliced)
- ½ C celery, cut in slices
- 1 3 oz. can mushrooms, sliced
- 1 T sugar
- ½ C broth
- 2 t corn starch
- ¼ C soy sauce

Brown meat in hot fat. Add next 6 ingredients.

Cover and simmer 5 minutes. Blend corn starch with 1 T water and soy sauce; add to meat, cook and stir until thick.

Serve with rice and Chinese noodles. 4 to 5 servings.

ORIENTAL SHORTRIBS

- 4 lbs. short ribs well trimmed
- 3 cloves of garlic, minced
- ⅓ C soy sauce
- ⅓ C honey
- ⅓ C water

Coat ribs well with flour. Brown on all sides in oil, add garlic and brown. Pour off excess fat. Mix soy sauce, honey and water. Add to meat and cover. Taste for salt.

Bake 1½ to 2 hours at 350 degrees.

CHINESE BEEF & PEA PODS

- 1½ lb sliced sirloin steak
- 1 T oil
- ½ lb bean sprouts
- 1 pkg. frozen pea pods, thawed
- ½ C chopped green onions
- 1 can consommé
- 3 T soy sauce
- 1½ T corn starch
- 2 T water
- salt to taste

Brown meat slices in oil, remove from skillet. Cook bean sprouts, pea pods and onions in skillet for a few minutes, add consommé and soy sauce. Stir in corn starch that has been mixed with water. Cook and stir until clear and thickened. Add meat and mix well. Add salt if necessary. Serve over rice.

BROILED MARINATED FLANK STEAK

- 2 C red wine
- 1 C chopped onions
- 1 clove garlic, minced
- 1 bay leaf
- 1 large flank steak

Combine first four ingredients, place steak in shallow pan and add marinade. Marinate steak at least four hours or over night, turning steak occasionally.

Before broiling, remove steak from marinade and dry. Broil 5 minutes, sprinkle with salt and pepper and broil 5 minutes on other side. Slice diagonal slices and serve on heated platter.

ALL-IN-ONE SWISS STEAK

- 1 ½ lbs. round steak
- flour, salt and pepper
- 1 medium onion, sliced
- ½ green pepper, cut in strips
- 1 t Worcestershire sauce
- 2 lg. potatoes, sliced
- 1 can consommé
- 1 C water plus 2 T ketchup

Cut meat into 1/2 inch by 3 inch strips. Dredge with flour, salt and pepper. Brown in shortening, add the rest of ingredients, except potatoes. Simmer for about 45-50 minutes or until tender. Add sliced potatoes, adjust seasoning and simmer until potatoes are tender.

BEEF STROGANOFF

- 1 ½ lbs. sirloin tip steak cut into 3 inch lengths
- 1 medium onion, chopped
- salt and pepper
- 1 C sour cream
- 1 4 oz. can mushroom slices, undrained
- ½ C dry white wine
- ½ can cream of mushroom soup, undiluted

Sauté beef in oil until well browned. Add onions and sauté for about 5 minutes. Add salt and pepper. Add wine and soup and stir until well blended. Cook uncovered on low heat, stirring often, until meat is tender. Add mushrooms. Lower heat to lowest degree and stir in sour cream. Adjust seasoning. Serve with rice or broad noodles.

BAKED CHICKEN

- 2½ - 3 lb. cut up chicken
- 1 C bisquick
- 1 egg
- salt and pepper
- ¼ t ground garlic
- ¼ t paprika

Rinse and dry chicken pieces. Beat egg slightly, add about 1 T water and a little salt. Into a plastic bag, add the other ingredients. Dip the chicken pieces into egg mixture, then shake each piece separately in bag to coat well. Melt some shortening on a cookie sheet and place chicken pieces so that they do not touch. Bake 70 minutes 350 degrees or until brown and crisp.

ITALIAN STYLE CHICKEN

- 2½ - 3 lb. fryer, cut in serving pieces
- 1 onion
- 2 cloves garlic, minced or crushed
- 6 oz. can tomato Juice
- 4 oz. can button mushrooms
- salt and pepper
- 1½ C spaghetti sauce

Lightly brown seasoned chicken in oil, add onion, juice and garlic. Cover and cook about 35 minutes or until chicken is tender.

About 5 minutes before serving, pour 1 C spaghetti sauce and mushrooms over chicken. Heat and serve with spaghetti. Garnish with sliced green or black olives.

STUFFED BONELESS CHICKEN

- 2 C well-seasoned bread dressing
- 4 chicken breasts, boned
- 2 T melted margarine or butter
- salt, pepper, paprika
- ½ C dry white wine
- 1 can cream of chicken soup

Flatten chicken breasts. Place 1/2 C dressing molded in a mound, on a well-greased cookie tin. Place chicken breast over dressing. Sprinkle with salt, pepper and paprika and bake for 1 hour 350 degrees. Heat soup with wine, stirring constantly over low heat. Pour over chicken before serving.

CHICKEN LOAF

- 1 C macaroni, cooked and drained
- 1 C diced cooked chicken
- 1 C bread crumbs
- 1 ½ C warm milk
- ½ C grated process cheese
- ¼ C chopped green pepper
- 2 T chopped onion salt and pepper
- 3 eggs, beaten

Mix all ingredients together, season to taste. Bake in greased loaf pan for 1 hour at 325 degrees.

Serve with condensed cream of mushroom or chicken soup.

CHICKEN CHOP SUEY

- 2 C cut cooked chicken
- 3 T oil
- 1 C chicken broth
- ½ C sliced water chestnuts
- ½ C bamboo shoots, sliced
- 1 C celery sliced
- 1 C onion, chopped
- 3 T soy sauce
- 1½ T cornstarch
- 2 T water
- Chinese dried noodles
- ½ C chopped walnuts or cashews

Cook onions and celery in oil for a few minutes, add water chestnuts, bamboo shoots. Cook 2 to 3 minutes, then add broth and soy sauce. Mix corn starch and water and add, stirring until thickened. Add chicken. Add salt if needed. To serve, place noodles on plate, add chicken mixture.

Sprinkle with nuts. Serve with plain or fried rice on the side.

CHICKEN SUPREME

- 4 boned chicken breasts
- 4 slices boiled or baked ham
- 4 T butter or margarine
- 2 T parsley
- ½ C sliced green or black olives
- 1 can cream of chicken soup
- ½ C white wine

Flatten chicken breasts; cream butter or margarine with parsley, spread inner side of chicken with butter mixture. Place slice of ham on top of butter and roll and tie each chicken breast. Sprinkle with salt and pepper and place in greased shallow baking pan. Place in 375 degrees for 15 minutes. Lower oven to 350 degrees. Blend soup and wine and pour over chicken with olives, cover and bake for 30-35 minutes more.

CHICKEN LIVERS IN WINE SAUCE

- 1 lb. chicken livers cut in thirds
- 1 lg. onion, sliced thin
- ¼ C water
- ½ C dry red wine
- 3 oz. can cut mushrooms

Mix about ½ C flour, salt, pepper in plastic bag. Shake livers to coat well. Lightly brown onions in oil, add livers and simmer. Covered for about 5 minutes. Add wine, water, mushrooms and juice. Taste for proper seasoning.

Heat for about 5-7 minutes. Serve over rice. Garnish with green peas.

ROAST LOIN OF PORK

- 3 ½ lb. boneless pork loin
- 3 T butter or margarine
- salt and pepper
- 1/8 t each rosemary, thyme, marjoram, garlic powder

Remove most of the fat with a sharp knife. Mix butter or margarine with herbs and spices. Rub into meat getting into any slits the meat may have. Place on aluminum foil, bake in a slow oven 320 degrees about 1-3/4 hours. Remove from oven, let stand about 10 minutes, then slice thin. Return to pan, cover with foil and heat before serving.

BAKED CREOLE PORK CHOPS

- 4 to 6 loin or rib pork chops
- 8 oz. can tomato sauce
- 1 onion, sliced
- ½ C celery, sliced
- ½ green pepper, sliced
- ¼ C water
- salt, pepper and garlic powder

Brown pork chops in small amount of shortening. Place in baking dish. Mix remaining ingredients and add to chops. Adjust seasoning, cover and bake 30-35 minutes, 325 degrees.

BOILED DINNER

- 2 ½ to 3 lbs. brisket or corned beef
- 1 medium head cabbage
- 6 large carrots
- 6 potatoes, whole
- 1 can small whole beets

Cook meat until tender (about 2-1/2 hours) add potatoes, cabbage, cut in large pieces and carrots. Cook for 15 minutes more. Remove meat and slice. Serve meat, cabbage, potatoes, carrots and beets on each plate. Pass mustard or horseradish sauce.

GLAZED CORNED BEEF

- 4 lb. corned beef brisket

Cook brisket as directed on package. Remove corned beef from water, place in shallow baking pan and cover with glaze. Bake in 350 degrees for 30 minutes, basting with sauce several times. Cut in ¼ inch slices.

DRESSING

- ⅓ C chili sauce
- ⅓ C brown sugar
- 2 T lemon juice or vinegar
- 2 T prepared mustard

Mix well and baste corned beef several times during baking.

STUFFED BREAST OF VEAL

- 3 ½ - 4 lb. breast of veal
- bread stuffing
- salt, pepper, garlic

Have butcher cut a pocket in veal. Rub meat inside and out with seasonings. Stuff cavity loosely with dressing.

Skewer opening. Roast uncovered for 1 hour at 350 degrees then uncover and continue roasting for another 40 minutes or until meat is tender.

VEAL PARMIGIANA

- Thin boneless Veal steaks, (4 servings)
- 1 egg
- bread crumbs (seasoned)
- 1 lb. can marinara sauce
- 4 large slices mozzarella cheese
- Parmesan cheese, grated

Season veal steaks with salt and pepper, dust with flour. Beat egg plus 1 T water. Dip meat into egg mixture, then bread crumbs. Brown veal in oil about 2 minutes on each side. Place in greased baking pan. Place slice mozzarella cheese on each steak, then cover with sauce. Bake about 25 minutes 325 degrees. Sprinkle with Parmesan cheese and return to oven for 3 minutes more.

AMERICAN STYLE CASSOULET

- ½ lb. sweet Italian sausage
- 1 ½ lb. boneless lean pork
- 3 chicken breasts, skinned and boned
- 1 large onion, chopped
- clove garlic, minced
- 2 1-lb. cans cannellini beans
- 2 C dry white wine
- 3 beef bouillon cubes

Cut meat and chicken into cubes. Brown sausage in skillet, drain off most of the fat. Add pork, chicken, onion and garlic, salt and pepper. Cook until not quite brown. Stir in beans, wine and more salt if necessary. Place in 3 qt. casserole. Cover and bake about 1½ - 2 hours. Makes about 8 servings.

Serve with hot crusty French bread and butter.

BARBECUED LAMB

- 1 ½ - 2 lbs. lean lamb
- about 1 c barbecue sauce
- salt, pepper and garlic powder

Trim meat and cut into large chunks. Sprinkle with salt, pepper and garlic powder. Cover generously with sauce.

Place in open roasting pan and roast for about 40-45 minutes for 375 degrees or until meat is fork tender. Baste several times while meat is roasting. Serves 4.

SALMON LOAF

- 1 - 16 oz. can salmon, drained
- 1 T butter or margarine
- 1 C bread crumbs
- 1 C hot milk
- 2 eggs, well beaten
- salt & pepper

Remove all bones and skin from fish, mash well. Mix butter with hot milk and add to bread crumbs. Add well beaten egg, salt and pepper. Turn into greased 9X5 loaf pan. Bake 45-50 minutes in a 350 degrees oven.

Serve with rich white sauce, sprinkle with parsley.

FILLET OF SOLE

- 2 lbs. fillet of sole
- salt and pepper
- paprika and lemon juice

Spread aluminum foil in pan and place fillets so they do not touch. Sprinkle with seasoning and lemon juice. Place about 1 T butter on each slice. Place under broiler for about 5-6 minutes.

BAKED HALIBUT

- 1 ½ lbs. halibut, fresh or frozen
- 2 cans stewed tomatoes
- 1 onion, chopped
- salt and pepper

Cook onion in margarine until tender, but not browned.

Add the stewed tomatoes, simmer for 2 minutes. Pour over fish, which has been sprinkled with salt and pepper. Bake for 35 minutes at 350 degrees. Fish should flake when tested with fork. Serves 4.

Casseroles & Pastas

A little of this and that, add some sauce, rice or pasta and there you have it, a casserole.

The combinations are limitless.

Here are a few starters.

NOODLE PUDDING

- 8 oz. medium noodles, cooked
- 2 eggs
- ½ C sugar
- ½ t cinnamon
- ¼ t salt
- 1 C cottage cheese
- 1 C sour cream
- 1 t lemon rind

Beat together, well; eggs, sugar, salt and cinnamon. Stir in cottage cheese, lemon rind and sour cream. Stir in noodles and blend well. Pour into 1½ qt. casserole

Bake 40-45 minutes 350 degrees. Serve with fruit sauce.

FRUIT SAUCE

- 1 lb. can fruit cocktail
- 1 ½ T sugar
- 2 t cornstarch
- ½ t lemon juice

Drain fruit, add corn starch, lemon juice and sugar to fruit syrup. Cook stirring constantly until mixture thickens and boils. Add fruit and cook for 5 minutes. Serve warm over pudding.

SPANISH NOODLES

- 8 oz. noodles, medium
- 2 onions, chopped
- 1 green pepper, chopped
- 1 clove garlic, minced or crushed
- 1 T shortening
- 1 lb. ground beef
- ½ C chopped or sliced black olives
- 2 T chili
- dash of thyme, salt, pepper and oregano
- 8 oz. can tomato sauce
- 1 lb. 13 oz can of small red beans
- ¾ C bread crumbs
- ½ C shredded Jack cheese

Fry onions, green pepper and garlic for a few minutes, add meat, crumble with fork. Add spices, tomato sauce and liquid from beans, simmer 10 minutes. Add noodles, beans and olives. Pour mixture in large casserole dish. Sprinkle with bread crumbs and cheese. Bake 25 minutes in 350 degrees.

NOODLES ROMANOFF

- 8 oz. noodles
- 1 pint cottage cheese
- 1 C sour cream
- 1 small onion, chopped
- 1 t salt
- 1 C shredded yellow cheese
- 1 C bread crumbs

Cook noodles in salted water and drain. Combine onion, cottage cheese and sour cream; add to noodles, season to taste. Place in 1-1/2 qt. greased casserole. Mix yellow cheese with crumbs, sprinkle over noodle mixture. Dot with margarine. Bake 350 degrees 35 minutes.

STUFFED SHELLS

- ½ package frozen chopped spinach, thawed
- ½ lb. creamed cottage cheese or ricotta
- salt
- 1 jar spaghetti with meat sauce
- ½ lb. ground beef
- ½ C dry red wine
- 8 oz. package large shells (pasta)
- Parmesan cheese

Cook shells in salted water and drain. Crumble and brown meat, add salt and pepper, drain fat, add sauce and wine and simmer about 5 minutes. Drain spinach and chop. Add cheese and salt. Fill shells with the mixture, place in shallow baking dish, cover with sauce. Sprinkle with Parmesan and bake 25-30 minutes.

MACARONI & CHEESE

- 2 ½ C uncooked macaroni
- processed cheese, cut in small chunks
- ¼ C margarine or butter
- 2 T flour
- 1 ⅓ C milk
- dash of pepper

Cook macaroni in salted water until just slightly tender, drain. Melt margarine, add flour and blend, gradually add milk stirring constantly, then add the cheese and pepper, stirring until cheese melts. Pour cheese sauce over macaroni. Mix until well coated. Pour into a well-greased casserole. Bake about 35 minutes 350 degrees or until brown around edges.

ENCHILADA PIE

- 3 Tortillas
- 1 lb. ground beef
- ½ onion, chopped
- salt
- ¾ t chili powder
- 6 oz. can tomato sauce
- ½ C sliced black olives
- 6 oz. water
- grated cheddar or Jack cheese

Brown meat, onions, add seasonings, sauce and olives. Using a 1½ qt. greased casserole, place one tortilla, meat sauce, cheese; repeat layers. Add water.

Bake covered for 25 minutes 350 degrees.

FRANKS AND KRAUT

- 1 onion, sliced thin
- 1 large can sauerkraut
- 8 all-beef frankfurters
- 8 strips of bacon, partially fried
- 4 slices process cheese caraway or dill seeds

Cook onion until tender but not brown. Add about 1 t of either seeds. Mix with sauerkraut and put in baking pan. Meanwhile, slit frankfurters lengthwise but not through. cut each slice of cheese in half and fold. Insert the cheese in slits. Wrap a slice of bacon around each frankfurter and place on sauerkraut. Bake at 375 degrees for 25 minutes. Delicious served with home fried potatoes and green vegetables.

LAYERED CASSEROLE

- 1 lb. ground beef
- 1 C cooked rice, salted
- 12 oz. can whole kernel corn
- 8 oz. can tomato sauce with onions
- salt, pepper, chili powder

Crumble and brown meat, drain most of fat. Add salt and pepper and ½ t chili powder. In a 2 qt. casserole place the rice, sprinkle with chili powder, then add meat, pour ½ can tomato sauce over meat, add corn and pour the rest of the tomato sauce. Cover and bake 30-35 minutes for 350 degrees.

CHICKEN RICE CASSEROLE

- 1 Frying chicken, cut up
- or about 2 lbs. of favorite parts
- 1 C water
- 1 package chicken-flavored rice
- 1 lb. can stewed tomatoes
- 1 package frozen peas, cooked

Rinse and dry chicken parts, brown in oil, drain off excess oil. Add water and envelope of seasoning from rice mix.

Add stewed tomatoes. Cover and simmer for about 20 minutes. Meanwhile brown rice in margarine. Stir into sauce in pan with chicken. Cover and simmer for about 25-30 minutes until chicken is tender. Serve mound of rice with peas on top and chicken on the side.

BEAN CASSEROLE

- 1½ lbs. ground beef
- 2 t salt
- ¼ t garlic powder
- 1 t chili powder
- 6 oz. bag corn chips
- 1 medium onion, chopped
- 2 cans refried beans (1 lb. 4oz.)
- 1 can or pkg. enchilada sauce
- 1 C grated cheese (cheddar or jack)

Brown meat, drain; add salt, garlic, chili. Mix together beans, onions and enchilada sauce. Stir in meat and half the corn chips crushed. Place in 2½ qt. casserole, circle with remaining chips. Bake 30 minutes. Sprinkle with cheese. Bake 10 minutes longer.

CHICKEN CASHEW CASSEROLE

- 1½ C cooked chicken, cut in chunks
- 1 small can mandarin oranges, drained
- 1 C celery, sliced
- ½ C onion, chopped
- 1 can condensed cream of mushroom soup
- ¼ C water or chicken broth
- 13 oz. can Chinese dry noodles
- ½ C cashew nuts

Cook celery and onions until barely tender, in oil. Combine all ingredients, except 1/2 c of noodles, in 2 qt. casserole. Sprinkle the remaining noodles on top. Bake for 30 minutes 325 degrees. Serve with white rice.

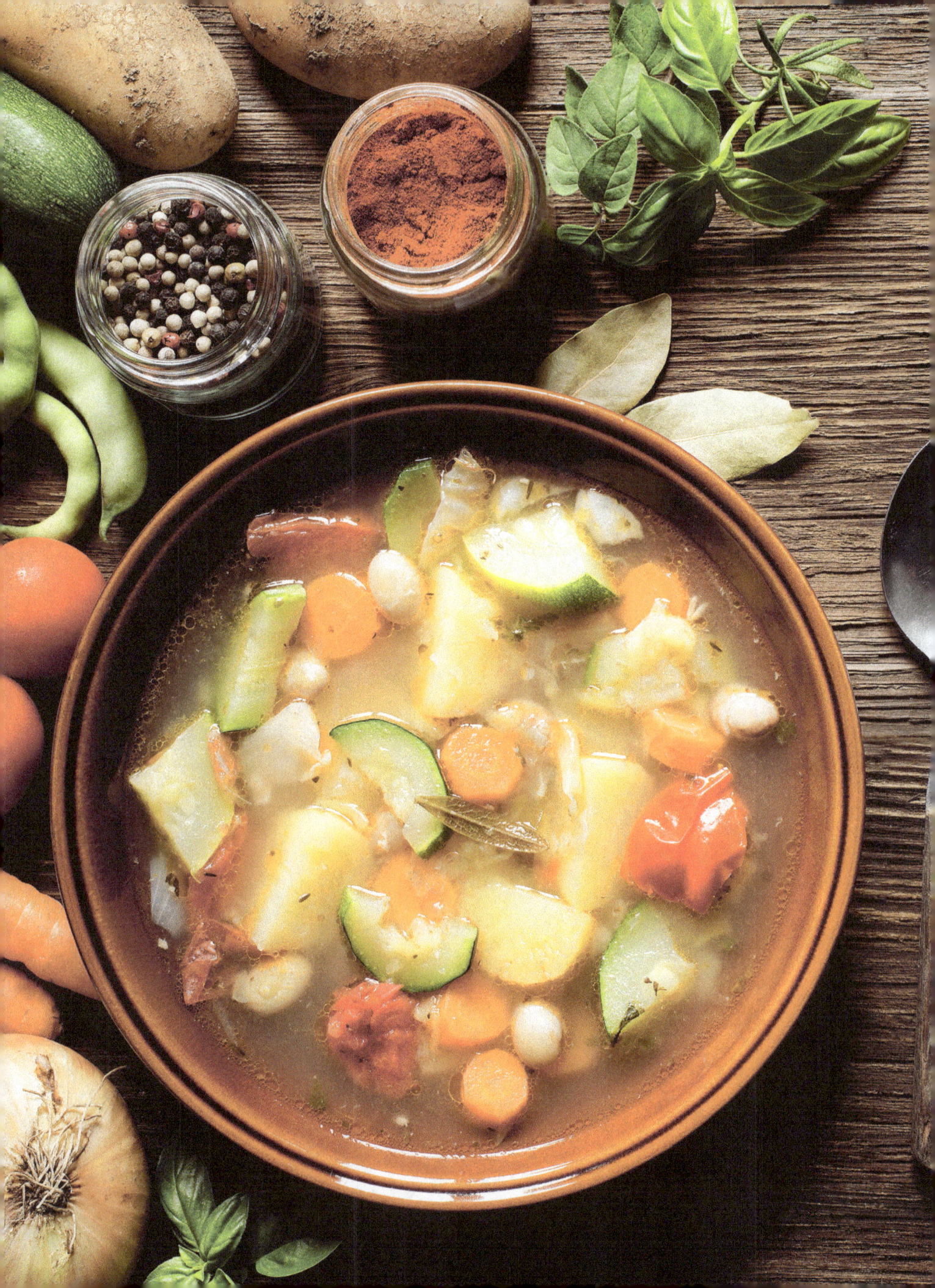

Vegetables & Soups

We are so fortunate to have the variety of vegetables in our markets year round.

Nutritionists say we should include at least two vegetables a day and vegetables are so good cooked with a little salt, or a squeeze of lemon juice. But like anything else good, we long for a change.

A little sauce or change of seasoning does the trick, a combination of two vegetables for variety helps. The combinations are endless. Be creative!!

A bowl of homemade soup can do so much for ones disposition, on a cold rainy day a bowl of hot soup can change our mood, it is my idea of "soul food".

Try making your own soup and freeze some for those hurried days.

SCALLOPED POTATOES

- 4 C thinly sliced potatoes
- ½ C chopped onions
- flour (about ½ C)
- 1 t salt pepper
- 2 T butter
- 1½ C hot milk

Arrange layer of potatoes in 2 qt. greased casserole, sprinkle with flour, salt & pepper. Dot with butter; repeat layers. Pour milk over all. Sprinkle with paprika. Cover, bake 45-55 minutes, or until potatoes are tender.

STUFFED BAKED POTATOES Version 1

- 4 large Idaho potatoes
- 4oz. can slice mushrooms, drained
- 1 C white sauce
- salt and pepper

Bake potatoes; cut in half and remove potato, leaving skins intact. Mash with half or white sauce; salt and pepper.

Place potato mixture back in skins and pour mushrooms, mixed with other half cup of white sauce, over potatoes. Put back in oven and heat for 10-15 minutes.

STUFFED BAKED POTATOES Version 2

- 4 large Idaho or russets, baked and cut in halves
- 4 strips of bacon, fried crisp and crumbled
- ½ C shredded mild cheddar cheese
- butter or margarine

Remove potato from skins and reserve skins. Mash potatoes with butter and about 2 T milk. Beat until fluffy.

Mix in bacon. Return to skins and top with cheese. Put under broiler for 2-3 minutes until cheese melts.

POTATOES IN CELERY SAUCE

- 5 potatoes, cooked and sliced thick
- 1 can condensed cream of celery soup
- ½ C milk
- ½ C bread crumbs
- ½ C grated, American, cheddar or Jack cheese
- salt and pepper
- chopped parsley

Add milk to soup, stirring until smooth, add potatoes, parsley and adjust seasoning. Pour into 1½ qt. casserole. Mix crumbs with cheese and top the potato mixture. Dot with margarine and bake 25-30 minutes in 350 degrees oven.

POTATO PANCAKES

- 2 c grated raw potatoes
- 2 eggs
- 1¼ t salt
- pepper
- 2 T flour or matzoh meal
- ½ onion, grated
- pinch of baking powder
- oil

Combine all ingredients except oil. Mix well. Heat oil in skillet, drop mixture by spoonfuls into hot oil. Fry until golden on both sides. Serve hot with apple sauce or sour cream. 4-6 servings.

FOR POTATO PUDDING

Pour mixture into well-greased casserole, spreading evenly in pan. Bake 350 degrees 1 hour or until edges are crisp.

SWEET POTATO BALLS

- 1 C sweet potatoes
- 2 T butter or margarine
- ¼ t salt
- 1 T sugar
- 8 cooked prunes, cut in halves
- crushed corn flakes

Mash sweet potatoes with butter, salt and sugar. Wrap potatoes around ½ prune, forming small balls.

Roll balls in corn flakes. Bake at 350° on greased cookie sheet for 25 minutes.

SWEET POTATO CASSEROLE

- 1 large can sweet potatoes, drained
- 1 C apple sauce*
- 1 T sugar
- 1 t cinnamon
- 2 T butter or margarine

Mash potatoes, add rest of the ingredients and beat with fork until well mixed. Pour into greased casserole and sprinkle with 2 T brown sugar. Bake 30-35 minutes at 350 degrees.

*1 c crushed pineapple, drained, may be use in place of apple sauce.

FRIED CABBAGE AND POTATOES

- 1 small head of cabbage, shredded
- 1 large onion, sliced
- 5 medium potatoes, cooked and sliced

In a large skillet place about 2 T margarine, when melted, add onions and cabbage and stir fry. When cabbage and onions become limp and turn a golden brown, move to one side, or remove if skillet is too small, and add more margarine and potatoes, as they brown. Keep turning them; mix the cabbage and potatoes together. Add salt and pepper to taste.

HARVARD BEETS

- 2 t corn starch
- ⅓ C sugar
- ½ t salt
- ⅔ C vinegar
- ⅓ C water
- 3 C sliced beets, fresh or canned
- 1 T butter

Mix corn starch with sugar and salt. Stir in vinegar and water. Cook, stirring constantly until mixture is thickened and smooth. Add beets. Stir in butter.

STEWED TOMATO CAULIFLOWER

- 1 head cauliflower, about 3 C flowerets
- 1 large can stewed tomatoes
- ½ green pepper, chopped
- ½ onion, chopped bread crumbs, salt, pepper
- Italian seasoning, about ¼ t

Cook cauliflower flowerets in salted water until just slightly tender, do not overcook. Sauté onions and green pepper until tender. Add stewed tomatoes, salt, pepper and Italian seasoning. Bring to boil. Place cauliflower in a ½ qt. casserole, pour sauce over it. Sprinkle with crumbs, about 1 C. Dot with butter or margarine. Bake for 20 minutes 350 degrees or until bubbly. Zucchini squash may be substituted for cauliflower.

FRENCH FRIED CAULIFLOWER

- 1 head cauliflower
- salted water bread crumbs
- 1 egg
- 1 T water
- paprika

Separate cauliflower into flowerets and cook in boiling salted water until just tender, about 10 minutes.

Drain, cool and wipe dry. Dip pieces into dry bread crumbs, then into egg beaten with water. Roll again in bread crumbs. Fry in shallow oil heated to 375 degrees about 5 minutes or until golden brown. Drain on absorbent paper and sprinkle with paprika. Makes 4 to 6 servings.

BAKED LIMA BEANS

- 2 packages frozen Lima beans, cooked
- 1 medium onion, chopped
- 3 T margarine
- 2 T flour
- 1 lb. can tomatoes
- ¼ t garlic powder
- salt and pepper

Sauté onions in margarine; add flour and stir. Add tomatoes and seasoning, simmer until thickened, add drained beans.

Pour into casserole, sprinkle with Parmesan cheese and flavored bread crumbs. Cover and bake 30 minutes in 350 degrees oven. Remove cover and bake 8 minutes more.

STUFFED YELLOW SQUASH

- ½ C cooked rice
- ½ lb. ground beef
- 1 small onion, minced
- salt and pepper
- 6 oz. can tomato sauce
- 4 medium yellow squash

Brown meat with onion, salt and pepper. Add tomato sauce and rice. Cut squash into halves, lengthwise, scoop out seeds, sprinkle with salt. Spoon mixture into centers of squash. Place in greased baking dish, cover and bake until tender 370 degrees about 25 minutes.

SQUASH MEDLEY

- 2 zucchini squash
- 2 summer squash
- 2 yellow crook neck squash

Wash and cut squash in slices. Cook in salted water. When tender serve with lump of butter or cream sauce.

CHINESE GREEN BEANS

- 2 packages cut style green beans, frozen
- 8 oz. can water chestnuts, drained and sliced
- 1 can cream of celery soup
- 2 4-oz. cans mushroom pieces, undrained
- ½ C sliced green onions
- salt

Cook beans until barely tender, drain. Add rest of the ingredients. Place in 2 qt. casserole. Bake 30 minutes 350 degrees. Remove from oven and top casserole with Chinese noodles or French fried onion rings. Return to oven and bake 5 minutes more.

CORN PUDDING

- 3 eggs
- 1 T sugar
- 1 t salt
- pepper (white)
- 1 lb. can whole kernel corn with pepper and pimento
- 2 C liquid from corn (add milk to make 2 cups
- 2 T margarine

Beat eggs well; add the rest of ingredients, except margarine. Pour into shallow casserole. Cut margarine and dot top of casserole. Bake 350 degrees 35-40 minutes or until set.

CORN OYSTERS

- ½ C flour
- 1 t salt
- ¼ t accent
- 2 C drained whole corn
- 2 eggs, separated

Sift together flour, salt and accent. Mix corn with egg yolks. Stir into flour. Beat egg whites stiffly, fold into corn mixture. Drop by spoonfuls in hot oil. Drain on paper towel.

STUFFED EGGPLANT

- 1 large eggplant
- 1 lb. ground beef
- ¼ C chopped onions
- ½ C grated Parmesan cheese
- 1½ C spaghetti sauce or tomato sauce that has been seasoned with onion and garlic

Slice eggplant, without peeling, about ½ inch thick; parboil in salted water for about 5 minutes. Remove slices carefully so as not to break them. Place a layer of slices in greased shallow baking pan. Meanwhile, crumble ground beef and brown; add salt, pepper and onions. Place meat in eggplant and cover with a layer of eggplant slices. Pour sauce over all and sprinkle with cheese. Bake 350 degrees for 30-35 minutes.

HAWAIIAN CARROTS

- 4 C sliced carrots
- 1 can pineapple chunks (1 lb. 4 oz.)
- salt
- 2 T butter or margarine

Cook carrots in pineapple juice, salt, butter and water. Simmer until tender. Add pineapple chunks and heat through. Nice served with pork roast.

STUFFED MUSHROOMS

- 16 large mushrooms ¼ lb. lean ground beef
- 2 T bread crumbs
- 1 egg yolk, beaten
- 1 T chopped onion salt and pepper

Chop mushroom stems. Crumble and brown ground beef, add onions, mushroom pieces, salt and pepper. Cool slightly, add egg yolk and bread crumbs. Fill mushroom caps very full. Bake for 15-20 minutes 375 degrees or broil for about 6-8 minutes.

FRIED RICE Version 1

- ½ C green onions, chopped
- 3 T oil
- ½ C sliced celery
- 1 C sliced mushrooms
- ¼ C sliced water chestnuts
- 3 C cold cooked rice
- 2 T soy sauce
- 1 egg slightly beaten

Sauté onions and celery in oil until tender, add mushrooms, water chestnuts and soy sauce, then rice. Mix gently with fork. Cook over low heat for 10 minutes. Add beaten egg and stir until egg is set.

FRIED RICE Version 1

- 3 C cold cooked rice
- 3 T oil
- ½ C chopped green onions
- 1 envelope Lipton onion soup mix
- 2 T soy sauce
- 1 beaten egg, fried and cut into small pieces
- ¼ C toasted slivered almonds
- ½ C browned pork, cut into small pieces

Stir soup mix into oil until blended, add rice and fork stir until well coated. Add meat, soy sauce then egg. Before serving sprinkle with chopped green onions and almonds.

RICE AND PEAS

- 2 C cooked white rice
- ½ stick margarine
- 1 package peas, thawed
- ¼ C sliced green onions
- salt and pepper

Mix all ingredients together and serve hot as side dish with beef roast or pot roast.

VEGETABLE BEAN SOUP

- 1 C Navy beans
- 1 Ham bone or 1 lb. soup meat and bone
- 1 medium onion
- 7 C water
- ½ C sliced celery
- salt, pepper and garlic powder
- 1 large potato, cubed
- 1 large carrot, sliced

Rinse beans, add water, bring to boil; simmer 2 minutes. Remove from heat and let stand for 1 hour. Add meat or ham, onion, salt, pepper and garlic powder. Cover and simmer

1 ½ hours or until beans are tender. Remove bone, onion and meat. Add vegetables and meat which have been cut into small pieces. Cook for 30 minutes more.

Taste for seasoning.

FRUIT SOUP

- 1 C dried apricots
- 1 C pitted prunes
- 5 C water
- 6 oz. can frozen orange juice
- ½ C sugar
- ½ lemon Cinnamon stick
- 2 T quick cooking tapioca

Combine fruits, water and juice. Let stand for 30 minutes. Add 1/2 lemon, cinnamon stick and sugar to fruit and simmer, covered, until almost tender. Taste; if needed, add more sugar or lemon to suit taste. Remove cinnamon stick. Serve cold with sour cream, topped with cinnamon or whipped cream.

DOUBLE CORN CHOWDER

- 1 large onion, chopped
- ½ green pepper, chopped
- 1 C diced potatoes
- 1 C sliced celery
- 1½ C milk
- 8 oz. can creamed corn
- 12 oz. can whole kernel corn
- sugar, salt, pepper and accent

Cook onion and green pepper until tender, but not browned. Add 2 cups of water, celery, potatoes, salt, pepper and a dash of accent. Simmer until potatoes are tender; add both cans of corn, milk and about 1 teaspoonful of sugar.

Adjust seasoning. Heat but do not boil. Serves 4-6.

BEAN SOUP

- 1 lb. soup meat and marrow bone
- 1 ½ C Navy or Pea beans
- 7 C water
- 1 onion
- 2 lg. stalks celery cut in small pieces
- 2 lg. carrots, diced
- 2 strips of bacon cut in small pieces
- 8 oz. can tomatoes, chopped
- Salt and pepper to taste
- dash of garlic powder

Put meat, bones, beans in water; add 1 t salt and cook 30 minutes.

Add onions and cook 1 hour, then add carrots, celery and tomatoes. Taste for seasoning, cook 30 minutes or until beans are very soft. Remove meat, cut into small pieces and return to pot.

POTATO-CORN SOUP

- 6 slices bacon
- 1 lg. onion, chopped
- 2 c chicken broth
- 2 C milk
- 2 C mashed potatoes
- 17 oz. can creamed corn
- salt and pepper to taste

Fry bacon until crisp; drain off fat, leaving about 2 T to fry onions. When onions are tender, add remaining ingredients. Heat again. Add crumbled bacon on top before serving.

POTATO LEEK SOUP

- 5 medium potatoes, diced
- 3 leeks, sliced, only the white part
- ½ C celery, sliced
- salt and pepper

Place all ingredients in soup kettle, add water and cover. Bring to boil, then lower flame and simmer until potatoes are very soft. Put vegetables through sieve or food mill. Add milk or light cream to thin. Garnish with chopped parsley.

MINESTRONE

- 6 C of beef or chicken broth
- 1 C shredded cabbage
- 1 pkg. frozen mixed vegetables, thawed
- 8 oz. can red kidney beans, drained
- 8 oz. can garbanzo beans, drained
- 1 lg. potato, diced
- 1 lg. onion, chopped
- ¼ t garlic powder
- salt and pepper
- 8 oz. can whole tomatoes, cut in small pieces, use liquid

Put ingredients together in a large soup kettle. Simmer for 40 minutes, adjust seasoning. Tiny meatballs may be added if desired.

BARLEY AND MUSHROOM SOUP

- 1 lb. short ribs, trimmed
- 1 lg. marrow bone
- 1 cCbarley
- 1 lg. onion
- 2 qts. water
- 2 carrots, sliced
- 2 stalks celery, sliced
- about 4-6 imported dried mushrooms
- salt and pepper
- dash of garlic powder

Place meat, bone and barley in kettle and cover with water. Bring to boil then lower flame and simmer for about 1½ hours or until meat is tender. Meanwhile wash mushrooms and soak in about 1/4 c water until pliable; cut into pieces, use mushroom liquid in soup. After meat is tender add the rest of the ingredients and season. Let cook for about 30-40 minutes more. Serves 4-6.

LENTIL SOUP

- 6 C water
- 1½ C lentils
- 1 large onion, whole
- ½ C celery, sliced
- ½ C carrots, grated
- salt and pepper
- 2-3 frankfurters, sliced

Soak lentils for 2 hours. Drain; combine all ingredients except frankfurters. Bring to a boil, lower heat and simmer for 50 minutes. Discard onion, add frankfurters and simmer for 10 minutes more.

FRANKFURTER CHOWDER

- 3 T butter
- 2 small onions, sliced
- 4 franks, sliced thick
- ½ small cabbage, shredded
- 2 cans condensed beef broth plus 2 cans water
- 1 clove garlic, crushed
- 2 medium potatoes, diced
- 3 lg. carrots, sliced
- 2 stalks celery, sliced
- salt and pepper to taste

Sauté onions and garlic. Add cut franks, cabbage, potatoes, celery, broth, water, salt and pepper. Simmer 30 to 40 minutes until potatoes are tender.

CHICKEN SOUP

- 2 lbs. chicken necks and backs + water to cover, about 7 cups
- 1 large onion
- 3 stalks of celery, cut in large pieces
- 2 carrots, diced parsley
- salt and pepper

Place chicken and water in soup kettle, add onion. Bring to boil then reduce flame and simmer for 25 minutes. Add rest of ingredients except parsley and continue cooking for 25 minutes more. Remove chicken, onion and celery. Cut meat from bones and return to soup; add parsley. Serve with noodles, rice or matzoh balls.

MEATBALL SOUP

- 1½ lbs. ground beef
- 1 egg
- ½ C soft bread crumbs
- ½ C water
- 1 t salt
- 1 bay leaf
- ½ t chili powder
- 2 T oil
- 4 C water or broth
- 2 beef cubes
- 1 onion, sliced
- 1 C celery, sliced
- 1 C carrots, sliced
- 2 C cabbage, shredded
- 1 6 oz. can tomato paste
- 1 t salt
- 1 lb. can kidney beans, undrained

Combine first 6 ingredients; shape into small balls. Brown in deep kettle in oil, drain fat. Add remaining ingredients except beans. Bring to boil; simmer, covered, 35 minutes.

Remove bay leaf and add beans the last 10 minutes of cooking. Makes 6 servings.

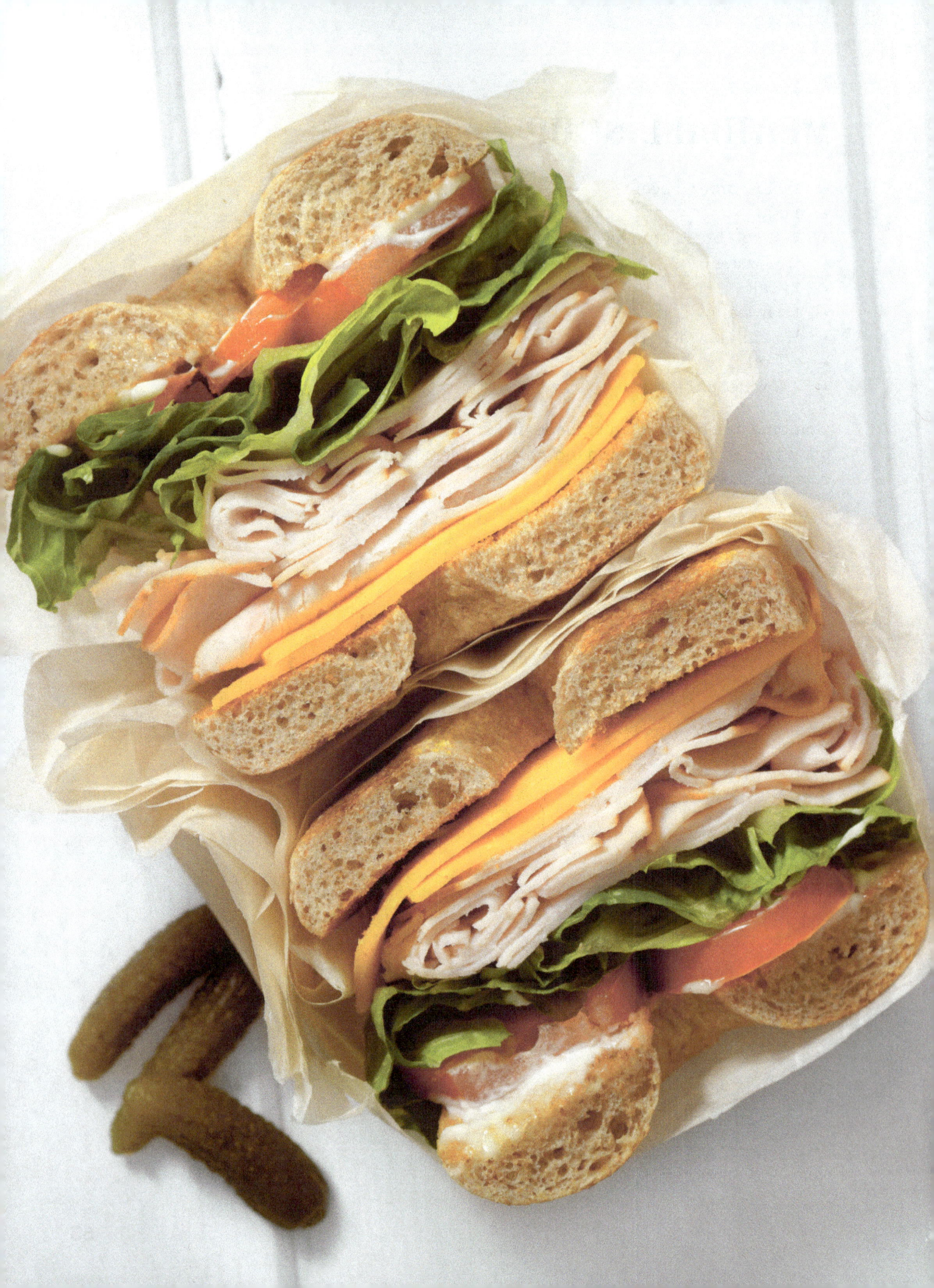

Sandwiches

Anything or a combination of almost anything between two slices of bread constitutes a sandwich. Surely we can do better than that.

To make a sandwich interesting try different breads and rolls.

Add a change of dressing or a combination of dressing.

The following are a few of our favorites.

GRILLED ROAST BEEF

- 8 slices rye bread
- 12 slices roast beef
- ketchup
- horseradish sauce

Spread ketchup on four slices of bread, add roast beef, then horseradish sauce. Cover with other slices of bread. Grill in margarine or butter. Serves 4.

FRENCH FRIED CHICKEN SALAD SANDWICH

- 8 slices egg bread
- 2 C chicken salad
- 1 egg, beaten
- ½ C milk

Place ½ C chicken salad on four slices of bread, cover with other slices. Beat egg slightly, add milk, and a dash of salt. Dip sandwiches in egg and milk mixture. Fry on both sides until golden brown. Serves 4.

CORN BEEF & COLE SLAW

- 8 slices rye bread
- 16 slices corned beef, sliced thin
- 1 C coleslaw
- mustard or Thousand Island salad dressing

Spread four slices with mustard or dressing. Add corned beef and top with ¼ c slaw to each sandwich. Cover with remaining bread slices. Serve with dill pickle spears. Serves 4.

UNITED NATIONS SANDWICH

- 2 round Armenian rolls
- 1 lb. can pork and beans
- 1 lb. can sauerkraut, drained and heated
- 4 kosher style knackwurst, cooked

Cut rolls in half, keeping bottoms and sides intact.

In roll opening, place mustard, ¼ C beans, 1 knackwurst split. Place on cookie sheet and heat in a preheated 400 degree oven for 5 minutes. Top with sauerkraut. Serves 4.

TURKEY & SALAMI SANDWICH

- 8 slices rye bread
- 8 slices white meat turkey
- 8 slices all beef salami, kosher style
- Thousand Island dressing
- lettuce

Spread dressing on four slices of bread and place 2 slices of salami and 2 slices of turkey on each slice. Spread more dressing on turkey, add lettuce and cover with other slices of bread. Makes 4 sandwiches.

OPEN COMBINATION SANDWICH

- 4 slices bread, any kind
- 1 C baked beans
- 8 slices bacon, crisp
- 4 slices processed cheese
- 4 lg. slices tomatoes

Spread each slice of bread with margarine or butter, add ¼ C baked beans, 1 slice of cheese, 2 slices of bacon and a slice of tomato. Put under broiler for 5 minutes, watching carefully so cheese does not burn. Serve hot. Serves 4.

CHILI SANDWICH

- 2 cans chili beef soup
- 4 lg. French or Italian rolls
- 1 C Jack cheese, shredded

Heat soup without adding water. Cut rolls and cover both sides with the chili mixture. Top with cheese and put in oven until cheese melts. Serve with tossed green salad for quick supper dish.

BANANA & CREAM CHEESE

- 8 slices raisin or cinnamon bread
- 2 bananas
- whipped cream cheese
- butter or margarine

Spread four slices of bread generously with whipped cream cheese, add 1/2 sliced banana to each, spread butter or mayonnaise on the four remaining bread slices and complete the sandwich.

BOLOGNA & CREAM CHEESE

- 8 slices pumpernickel bread
- 8 slices bologna
- whipped cream cheese

Spread 4 slices of bread generously with whipped cream cheese. Cover with bologna, add 2-3 thin slices of dill pickles. Cover with remaining slices of bread. Cut into quarters. Serves 4.

HAMBURGERS, 7 Ways

Allow ¼ lb. of good quality ground beef for each portion.

Try a variety of rolls and breads with the following recipes, such as:

- Sour dough
- Crusty French bread
- Toasted Italian or French rolls
- Rye bread
- Toasted English muffins
- Toasted cheese bread
- Egg rolls with sesame seeds

VERSION 1

Add 1/4 C pineapple juice to meat. Broil patties about 5 minutes, turn, place a pineapple slice on each patty and continue broiling for about 5 minutes more.

VERSION 2

Add ½ t Worcestershire sauce to meat. Wrap strip of bacon around patty. Add a thick slice of onion and tomato for last 2 minutes of broiling.

VERSION 3

Mash 1 medium avocado, add 1 T finely chopped onion, 1 small tomato, chopped fine, salt, pepper and garlic powder. Broil hamburgers. Before serving, place the avocado mixture on each patty.

VERSION 4

Add ¼ C chopped mushrooms to meat mixture and 1 T ketchup. Broil, serve with mushroom gravy.

VERSION 5

Place 1 T baked beans plus 1 T finely chopped onion in the center of half a patty. Cover with other half and seal edges. Broil.

VERSION 6

Add ½ C grated mild cheddar cheese to meat mixture. Broil and serve with cheese sauce.

VERSION 7

Add ¼ C grated Parmesan cheese and ½ t Pizza seasoning to meat mixture. Serve with Pizza sauce.

Cakes, Pies & Cookies

With everyone so diet conscious, perhaps I should have excluded this chapter. *NEVER!*

Life wouldn't be worthwhile if we didn't indulge, so cut smaller portions, don't apologize and enjoy yourself.

DEVILS FOOD CAKE

- ½ C margarine
- 1¼ C sugar
- 2 eggs
- 1 t vanilla
- 2 sq. unsweetened chocolate, melted
- 1¾ C flour
- ¾ t baking soda
- ½ t salt
- 1 C milk

Cream sugar and margarine together until fluffy. Add eggs, vanilla and beat until well blended. Add melted chocolate and blend. Combine dry ingredients and add alternately with milk. Pour into two greased 8 inch round layer cake pans.

Bake 350 degrees for 30 minutes or until done.

Frost with chocolate frosting. Decorate with chocolate curls, whole walnuts or chocolate shot.

APPLESAUCE CAKE

MIX THOROUGHLY:
- 1 C applesauce
- ⅞ C brown sugar
- ½ C oil

SIFT INTO LARGE BOWL:
- 1¾ C flour
- 1 t baking soda
- ½ t salt
- 1 t cinnamon
- ½ t cloves

add, 1/2 c chopped walnuts

Add the applesauce mixture. Blend well and pour into a greased 8 or 9 inch square baking pan. Bake at 350 degrees for 35-40 minutes. Cool. Frost if desired or sprinkle with confectioner's sugar.

CHOCOLATE STRUESEL COFFEE CAKE

- ⅔ C margarine or butter
- 1 C sugar
- 2 eggs
- 1½ t baking powder
- ¼ t salt
- 1 C sour cream
- Streusel topping (see below)
- 1 t vanilla
- 1 t grated orange peel
- 2 C flour
- ½ t baking soda
- 1 oz. melted unsweetened chocolate
- ¼ C chopped nuts

Cream margarine and sugar, add eggs. Mix in sour cream, vanilla and peel. Mix well: stir in dry ingredients. Pour into 10 inch tube pan. Drizzle melted chocolate over batter and swirl with fork. Top with streusel. Bake 50 minutes

350 degrees. Cool for 10 minutes in pan then lift out, leaving tube in cake. Cool on wire rack.

CHOCOLATE STRUESEL COFFEE CAKE

- ⅔ C margarine or butter
- 1 C sugar
- 2 eggs
- 1½ t baking powder
- ¼ t salt
- 1 C sour cream
- Streusel topping *(see below)*
- 1 t vanilla
- 1 t grated orange peel
- 2 C flour
- ½ t baking soda
- 1 oz. melted unsweetened chocolate
- ¼ C chopped nuts

Cream margarine and sugar, add eggs. Mix in sour cream, vanilla and peel. Mix well: stir in dry ingredients. Pour into 10 inch tube pan. Drizzle melted chocolate over batter and swirl with fork. Top with streusel. Bake 50 minutes

350 degrees. Cool for 10 minutes in pan then lift out, leaving tube in cake. Cool on wire rack.

STREUSEL TOPPING

- 5 T margarine
- ⅓ C brown or white sugar
- 1 egg yolk
- 1 C flour
- 2 t cinnamon

Cream margarine with sugar. Blend in egg yolk, flour and cinnamon. Mix with fork or pastry blender until crumbly.

SOUR CREAM APPLE CAKE

COMBINE and set aside:

- *½ C chopped walnuts*
- *½ C sugar*
- *2 t cinnamon*

- ½ C margarine
- 2 eggs
- 1 t vanilla
- 2 C flour
- 1 t baking powder
- ½ t salt
- 1 t baking soda
- 1 c sour cream
- 1 large tart apple, peeled and sliced thin

Beat at high speed, margarine, sugar, then add egg and vanilla. Beat until fluffy and light. Add dry ingredients alternately with sour cream. Spread half the batter in a well-greased 9 inch tube pan. Place apple slices around batter, sprinkle with half of nuts, sugar mixture; add rest of batter and sprinkle with remaining nut mixture. Bake 375 degrees 40 minutes or until done. Let cool on wire rack for about 30 minutes before lifting from pan.

ORANGE CRUNCH COFFEE CAKE

- 2 eggs
- 2 C biscuit mix
- ¼ c sugar
- ⅔ C milk
- ½ C chopped walnuts

Beat eggs well. Mix biscuit mix with sugar, add alternately with milk to beaten eggs. Stir in nuts. Spread in greased 8 inch pan. Bake 400 degrees 25 minutes. While cake is still warm, cover with topping (see below).

ORANGE TOPPING

Mix ⅓ C melted margarine with ⅔ C brown sugar.

Spread on warm cake. Sprinkle with ½ C chopped walnuts mixed with 2 T orange rind. Pour ½ C orange juice over mixture and place under broiler until bubbly. Serve warm.

FRUIT-TOP COFFEE CAKE

- 2 C flour
- 1 t salt
- 1 T baking powder
- ½ C sugar
- ⅓ C margarine
- 1 well beaten egg
- ⅓ C milk
- 1/3 C peach syrup
- 1 can sliced peaches

Cut margarine into dry ingredients until mixture resembles coarse crumbs. Combine egg, milk and syrup; add to flour mixture. Stir until just moistened. Spread in greased 8 inch square pan. Sprinkle with topping. Bake 350 degrees 45 minutes.

CRUNCHY TOPPING

Crush 2 C corn flakes, add ¼ C sugar, 1 t cinnamon and 2 T melted margarine. Mix together. After cake bakes, arrange peaches on cake and place in oven to heat through. Serve warm.

FILLED COFFEE CAKE

- 1/4 C margarine
- 1 C sugar
- 2 egg yolks
- 2 egg whites, stiffly beaten
- 1½ C flour
- 2 t baking powder
- ½ t salt
- 1 t vanilla
- ½ C milk

Cream shortening and sugar, add egg yolks. Mix well. Combine dry ingredients and add alternately with milk; add vanilla and fold in egg whites. Pour half the batter in greased 9 inch baking pan, sprinkle filling, cover with rest of batter. Bake 350 degrees 35 minutes or until top springs back when lightly touched.

FILLING

- ½ C brown sugar
- 1 T flour
- 1 t cinnamon
- 1 T melted shortening
- ¼ C chopped nuts

FRUIT COCKTAIL CAKE

- 1 C flour
- 1 C sugar
- 1 t baking soda
- 1 egg
- 1 lb. can fruit cocktail
- ¼ t salt
- ½ t vanilla

Mix all ingredients together including the juice from fruit. Pour into 8 inch greased baking pan. Sprinkle top with 2 T brown sugar and ¼ C chopped nuts. Bake 45-50 minutes 350 degrees.

SOUR CREAM BANANA CAKE

- ¼ C margarine
- 1⅓ C sugar
- 2 eggs
- 1 t vanilla
- 2 C flour
- 1 t baking powder
- 1 t baking soda
- ½ t salt
- 1 C sour cream
- 1 C mashed ripe bananas
- ½ C chopped nuts

Mix all ingredients together including the juice from fruit. Pour into 8 inch greased baking pan. Sprinkle top with 2 T brown sugar and ¼ C chopped nuts. Bake 45-50 minutes 350 degrees.

POPPYSEED CAKE

- 1 C shortening
- 1½ C sugar
- 1 12 oz. can poppy filling
- 4 eggs, separated
- 1 t vanilla
- 1 C sour cream
- 2½ C flour
- 1 t baking soda
- 1 t salt

Cream shortening and sugar until fluffy. Add poppy filling. Add egg yolks, one at a time, beating well after each one. Add vanilla and sour cream and blend. Add dry ingredients. Fold in, stiffly beaten, egg whites. Pour into a greased 9 or 10 inch tube pan. Bake 350 degrees 1 hour 15 minutes or until done. Cool for 5 minutes. Remove from pan. Decorate with confectioner's sugar.

FILLED CHIFFON CAKE

- 1 package lemon chiffon cake mix

Prepare as directed on package. Bake in tube pan. Place cake upside down on serving plate. Slice top from cake about 1 inch down. Cut down into cake 1 inch from outer edge and 1 inch from middle hole. Scoop out cake with spoon, being careful not to break sides or bottom. Fill and replace top (see fillings below). Frost with whipped cream or frosting.

VERSION 1
1 package instant chocolate pudding mix, using 1¾ C milk; let thicken before using for filling. Add ½ t vanilla and 1 T white rum.

VERSION 2
1 package instant vanilla pudding
1 C sweetened well drained sliced strawberries

VERSION 3
Any gelatin and fruit combination. When firm, whip and fold in ½ C whipped cream.

VERSION 4
2 cups whipped cream to which you may add: chopped sweetened fresh peaches, sweetened sliced strawberries, or sliced bananas.

VERSION 5
Lemon pie filling: Cook as directed on package. Cool before filling cake. Frost cake with fluffy white frosting and coconut.

CHIFFON CHEESECAKE

- 16 Zwieback, crushed
- 3 T sugar
- ¼ C melted shortening

Mix together, set aside ½ C; press remainder in 9 inch spring form.

- 3 C cottage cheese
- 3 eggs, separated
- ¼ C flour
- Juice and rind of 1 lemon
- 1 C whipped cream
- ¾ C sugar

Put cheese through sieve. Beat eggs with sugar until light and thick, add flour, salt, cheese, juice and rind. Mix well. Beat egg whites, add sugar and beat until stiff.

Fold into whipped cream then fold into cheese mixture. Pour into pan, sprinkle the rest of the crumbs. Bake 300 degrees 1¼ hours. Turn off heat, let stay in oven 45 minutes. Cool in pan.

GINGERBREAD SUPREME

- 1 package of Gingerbread mix
- 1 lb. jar applesauce
- ½ t cinnamon
- 8 coconut macaroons or cookies, crushed
- 1 cup whipped cream, sweetened

Bake gingerbread as directed on package. Cool.

Cover top with applesauce, then sprinkle with cookie crumbs; add cinnamon to whipped cream and top each portion with a generous dollop of whipped cream.

CHEESY-CAKE

- 1 8 oz. package cream cheese
- ⅔ C sugar
- ½ C sour cream
- 1 t vanilla
- 2 eggs

Cream first four ingredients well. Add eggs one at a time, beating well after each addition. Set aside.

- 1 C flour
- 1 t baking powder
- ½ t salt
- ½ C butter or margarine
- ⅔ C sugar
- 2 eggs
- 1 T milk
- 1 t vanilla

Cream butter or margarine with sugar, add eggs, beat well. Stir in milk and vanilla. Add the dry ingredients, which have been mixed together. Blend well. Pour into a well-greased 10 inch deep pie pan or a 9X9 sq. baking pan.

Spread batter over bottom and sides. Spoon cheese mixture over batter. Bake 325 degrees 40-45 minutes. Spread with topping and bake for 5 minutes more..

TOPPING

Combine 1 C sour cream, 2 T sugar, 1 t vanilla.

CHOCOLATE ROLL

- ¾ C sugar
- 4 stiffly beaten egg whites
- 4 egg yolks
- 1 t vanilla
- 6 T flour
- ¼ t salt
- ½ t baking powder
- 2 sq. unsweetened chocolate, melted

Fold sugar into beaten egg whites. Beat egg yolks until very light, add vanilla; Fold into stiffly beaten egg whites and sugar mixture; fold in dry ingredients. Stir in chocolate. Bake in waxed-paper lined 10X15 inch pan at 400 degrees 10-12 minutes. Turn out on cloth, sprinkled with confectioner's sugar. Trim edges. Roll with cloth and let stand until cool. Unroll and fill with Grasshopper filling. Roll again. Sprinkle with confectioner's sugar.

VARIATIONS:

1. Coffee whipped cream: add 1½ t instant coffee to whipped cream
2. Vanilla or Peach ice cream
3. Vanilla or Butterscotch pudding

PASTRY FINGERS

- ½ C dry cottage cheese
- ½ lb. butter
- 2 C flour
- ¼ t vanilla
- prune filling
- sugar

Combine sieved cheese, butter and flour. Blend with pastry blender. Knead slightly. Pinch off small pieces and form into balls the size of a walnut. Refrigerate overnight.

Roll each ball into 5 inch circles. Stir vanilla into filling. Place 1 T of filling in center of each circle. Roll and pinch ends. Bake on ungreased baking sheet 350 degrees 15 minutes. Sprinkle with sugar.

HUNGARIAN FRUIT SQUARES

- 3/4 C sugar
- 4 stiffly beaten egg whites
- 4 egg yolks
- 1 t vanilla
- 6 T flour
- ¼ t salt
- ½ t baking powder
- 2 sq. unsweetened chocolate, melted

Mix together: 3 T milk, 1½ t sugar, 1½ yeast.

Heat milk and sugar to lukewarm. Add yeast and set aside to rise. In a large bowl blend flour and butter with pastry blender, add baking powder. Make a well in center of mixture. Add slightly beaten egg yolks, sugar, vanilla and yeast mixture. Mix lightly. Form into 3 equal size balls.

Roll out first ball to size of pan approx. 9X13. Lift dough on rolling pin and place in pan. Spread with apricot filling. Roll out second ball and repeat the process using prune filling. Roll out third ball and cover second layer. Crimp the dough around pan. Cover and set aside to rise for about ½ hour. Bake 40 minutes at 350 degrees. Cool in pan for 5 minutes then invert. When cool cut in squares and sprinkle with confectioner sugar.

CHOCOLATE-CHERRY FRUITCAKE

- 3 eggs
- ¾ C sugar
- 1½ C flour
- 1½ t baking powder
- ¼ t salt
- 1 C chocolate chips
- 2 C chopped nuts
- 1 C raisins or chopped dates

Beat eggs, stir in sugar. Mix the rest of the ingredients together and add to egg and sugar mixture. Pour into paper lined greased 9X5X3 loaf pan. Place pan of water on bottom oven rack. Bake on top rack 350 degrees for 60 minutes.

Cool and remove from pan. Cool on rack.

PLAIN PASTRY

- 1¾ C flour
- 1 t salt
- ⅔ C vegetable shortening
- about ⅓ C ice water

Add shortening to flour and sprinkle water by tablespoonfuls. Stir with fork until dough forms a ball. Divide into 2 balls, wrap in wax paper and chill. Enough for two 8-9 inch pie shells or one 2 crust 9 inch pie.

Roll ball of dough on lightly floured canvas covered board. Roll from center towards edge, turning pastry several times. When it reaches 1 inch larger then pie pan, lift dough on rolling pin and gently place in pie pan. For 1 crust pie flute edges and prick bottom and side with fork. Bake 450 degrees 12 minutes.

APPLE PIE

- 6-7 C peeled sliced apples (Pippins or Gravensteins)
- ¾ C sugar
- 1 t cinnamon
- Pastry for 2 crust pie
- ¼ t nutmeg flour
- 1 t lemon juice butter

Mix all ingredients together, sprinkle about 2 T flour on mixture and stir to coat. Pile into unbaked 8-9 inch pie crust. Dot with butter. Cover with second crust or streusel. Bake 400 degrees 50-60 minutes.

APRICOT PRUNE PIE

- 2½ C mixed cooked dried fruit
- 1 T cornstarch
- ½ C sugar
- pinch of salt
- ¼ t cinnamon
- ½ C liquid from cooked fruit
- juice of 1 lemon
- 1 T butter

Mix corn starch with sugar, cinnamon and salt. Stir in liquid. Cook over low heat, stirring constantly until slightly thickened. Add lemon juice and butter, pour over fruit. Put fruit in unbaked pie crust, cover with remaining crust or lattice top. Crimp edges. If using full top, be sure to make slits for steam to escape. Bake 425 degrees for 30-35 minutes. Serve warm with whipped cream or vanilla ice cream.

LEMON MERINGUE PIE (9-inch pie)

- 1¼ C sugar
- ⅓ corn starch
- 1 C hot water
- ½ C milk
- 3 egg yolks, slightly beaten
- 3 T butter
- 5 T lemon juice
- grated lemon rind

Mix sugar and corn starch, add milk and water. Cook stirring constantly until mixture thickens and boils. Beat a small amount of hot mixture into eggs, return to saucepan and continue stirring. Boil for about 1 minute. Remove from heat, continue stirring while blending in butter, lemon juice and rind. Pour into baked pie shell. Cover with meringue being very careful to seal around the edges.

Sprinkle meringue lightly with sugar, also flaked coconut (optional). Place in oven. Bake 325 degrees until meringue is lightly browned..

MERINGUE

- 3 egg whites, at room temperature
- 1 T sugar

Beat until stiff, gradually adding about 1 T sugar. Continue beating until stiff peaks appear.

RHUBARB CREAM PIE

- 1 C sugar
- 3 T flour
- 1 t grated lemon peel
- 1 T butter
- 2 eggs
- 3 C cut rhubarb
- 1 recipe for 9 inch double pie crust

Blend sugar, flour, lemon peel and butter. Add eggs and beat smooth; pour over rhubarb. Pour into pastry lined pie pan. Top with pie crust. Bake 450 degrees 10 minutes then 350 degrees for about 30 minutes.

LEMON-ORANGE CHIFFON PIE

- 1 T unflavored gelatin
- ¼ C water
- ½ C plus 1 T sugar
- ⅓ C lemon juice
- 3 T orange juice
- 2 egg yolks
- ½ t salt
- 4 eggs
- 1 T grated lemon peel
- ¼ C sugar
- 4 egg whites
- 1 9-inch baked pie shell

Soften gelatin in cold water, combine sugar and lemon juice. Add salt to egg yolks and beat until thick, add juice mixture; beat well. Cook in double boiler until mixture coats spoon. Remove from heat, add softened gelatin and stir until dissolved, add lemon peel. Chill until partially set. Slowly beat ¼ C sugar into beaten egg white. Beat until stiff. Fold into custard and pour into pie shell. Chill until set. Top with thin layer of whipped cream if desired. Garnish with orange slices.

STRAWBERRY CREAM PIE

- 1½ pint strawberries
- ½ C sugar
- 1 package vanilla pudding
- 1 C heavy cream, whipped with 3 T sugar and ½ t vanilla
- 1 9-inch baked pastry shell

Prepare pudding according to directions on package, adding ¼ t vanilla. Cover with waxed paper and cool. Slice strawberries, add sugar. Save ½ pint of the best whole berries. Fold berries into vanilla pudding, pour into pie shell. Cover with whipped cream, garnish with whole strawberries. Chill several hours before serving.

SOUR CREAM APPLE PIE

- pastry for single 9 inch pie crust
- 1¼ C sugar
- ½ C flour
- 1 C sour cream
- ½ t vanilla
- ¼ t salt
- 2 C chopped apples
- 1 t cinnamon
- ¼ C margarine

Partially bake pie crust for 7 minutes at 350 degrees. Mix ¾ C sugar and 2 T flour, stir in sour cream, beaten egg, vanilla and salt. Beat until smooth. Stir in apples and pour mixture in shell. Bake 30 minutes 350 degrees. Top with crumbs using: ½ C sugar, 6 T flour, margarine and cinnamon. Bake 10 minutes longer.

PEAR ALMOND CRUNCH PIE

- 1 9-inch pie shell, baked
- 1 lg. can pear halves, drained
- 1 pkg. instant vanilla pudding
- ¼ t almond extract
- ½ C toasted chopped almonds
- ¼ C grapenuts
- whipped cream (optional)

Prepare pudding according to instructions on package, adding the almond extract. Line pie shell with pears. Cut side down, pouring pudding over pears. Mix almonds and grapenuts and sprinkle over pudding. Chill for several hours in refrigerator. Serve with whipped cream if desired.

ROCKY ROAD PIE

- 8 or 9 inch baked pie shell
- 1 package chocolate pudding mix
- ¾ C miniature marshmallows
- ½ C coarsely chopped nuts
- 1½ C whipped cream
- shaved chocolate or chocolate shot

Prepare pudding according to directions on package. Cover with waxed paper and cool slightly. Add marshmallows and nuts. Spread with sweetened whipped cream. Decorate with shaved chocolate or chocolate shot. Chill.

CHOCOLATE CHIP COOKIES

- ½ C margarine
- 1 egg
- ½ C white sugar
- ¼ C brown sugar
- 1 t vanilla
- ¼ t salt
- 1 C flour
- ½ t baking soda
- ½ C chopped nuts
- 6 oz. pkg. chocolate chips

Cream margarine, sugar, egg and vanilla until light and fluffy. Add dry ingredients, then nuts and chocolate chips. Drop by teaspoonfuls, on ungreased cookie sheet. Bake 8 - 10 minutes at 375 degrees. Cool on wire rack.

CHOCOLATE WALNUT WAFERS

- 2 oz. melted unsweetened chocolate
- ½ C shortening
- 1 C sugar
- 2 eggs, well beaten
- 1 C chopped walnuts
- ¼ t salt
- ½ t vanilla
- ⅔ C flour

Cream shortening, sugar and eggs until fluffy. Stir in chocolate. Add nuts, salt, vanilla and flour. Mix well. Drop by teaspoonfuls on greased cookie sheet. Bake about 10 minutes at 350 degrees. Remove cookies carefully as they are very soft. Store covered with waxed paper between layers. If a crisper cookie is desired, store in loosely covered container.

BUTTER BALLS

- ½ C butter
- ½ C shortening
- 1 t vanilla
- 2 C flour
- 1 C chopped pecans
- 6 T confectioner's sugar

Cream butter and shortening; add vanilla, stir in flour and nuts. Mix well. Wrap in waxed paper and chill for about an hour. Shape into small balls, place on ungreased cookie sheet. Bake 400 degrees 10 minutes. Roll in confectioner's sugar while still warm. Flavor improves when stored for a day before serving.

CHOCOLATE COCONUT SQUARES

- 1 stick margarine
- 1 C graham cracker crumbs
- 1 C flaked coconut
- 6 oz. pkg. chocolate chips
- 1 C chopped nuts
- 1 can condensed milk

Melt 1 stick margarine in 9 inch square pan. Pour in 1 C graham cracker crumbs, then 1 C flaked coconut. Add chocolate chips and chopped nuts. Pour condensed milk over the mixture. Bake 30 minutes 350 degrees. Cool and cut into small squares.

CHOCOLATE NUT BARS

- ½ C margarine
- ½ t almond extract
- ¾ C confectioner's sugar
- 1 egg
- 2 sq. chocolate, melted
- ¾ C chopped walnuts
- 2 C flour
- ½ t salt

Cream margarine, extract and sugar; add egg, chocolate and beat well. Stir in nuts. Add dry ingredients. Mix well and pack in 8X8 inch pan. Cover with waxed paper and chill overnight. Cut in bars, bake on ungreased cookie sheet 375 degrees 10-12 minutes. Roll in sugar while warm.

BUTTERSCOTCH ALMOND COOKIES

- ½ C margarine
- 1 egg
- ¼ C white sugar
- 6 T brown sugar
- ½ t almond extract
- ½ t vanilla
- 1 C flour
- ½ t baking soda
- ½ C chopped toasted almonds
- ½ pkg. butterscotch chips

Cream margarine, sugar, egg and flavorings until light and fluffy. Add dry ingredients, mix well, then add nuts and chips. Drop by teaspoonfuls on ungreased cookie sheet.

Bake 8-10 minutes 375 degrees. Cool on wire rack.

COCONUT OATMEAL

- ½ C margarine
- 1 C brown sugar
- 1 egg
- 1 t almond extract
- 1 C flour
- ½ t baking powder
- ¼ t salt
- ½ t baking soda
- ½ C oatmeal
- 6 oz. flaked coconut

Cream margarine and sugar until light and fluffy. Add egg and almond extract, blend well, then add dry ingredients and mix well before adding oatmeal and coconut. Drop by teaspoonfuls. Bake 375 degrees 10-12 minutes.

POPPYSEED COOKIES

- ¼ lb. poppyseeds
- ½ C sugar
- ½ t salt
- ½ C shortening
- 2 ½ C flour (approx.)
- 2 t baking powder
- 2 eggs
- juice from 1/2 lemon
- sugar and cinnamon, mixed

Mix all ingredients together well. Add flour if dough is not stiff enough to roll. Roll dough very thin. Cut with cookie cutter. Sprinkle with sugar and cinnamon. Bake 375 degrees for about 12 minutes or until edges are brown.

LEMON COOKIES

- 1½ C flour
- ½ t baking powder
- ¼ t salt
- 1 C sugar
- ¾ C margarine or butter
- 1 egg plus 1 yolk
- 1 T grated lemon rind
- 3 T lemon juice

Cream margarine, sugar, egg and yolk, lemon rind and juice together until fluffy; add dry ingredients and blend well. Make small balls, place on greased cookie sheet. With bottom of a glass, which has been buttered, press balls until about ⅛ inch thick. Sprinkle with sugar. Bake 375 degrees about 12-15 minutes. Cool on rack.

THUMBPRINT COOKIES

- 1 C margarine
  (optional: use part butter)
- ½ C brown sugar
- 2 egg yolks
- 1 t vanilla
- 2 C flour
- ¼ t salt
- ¾ C finely chopped nuts

Mix first four ingredients together until well blended, add flour and salt. Roll into 1 inch balls. Dip into slightly beaten egg whites. Roll in nuts. Place on ungreased cookie sheet. Bake 5 minutes 375 degrees. Remove from oven quickly, press thumb or tip of teaspoon on top of each cookie. Return to oven and bake for 8 minutes longer. Cool and place in dents, jelly and half of candied cherry. You may also place 2 chocolate chips in center but do this just before removing cookies from oven.

SPRITZ

- 1 c soft butter
- ⅔ C sugar
- 3 egg yolks
- 1 t vanilla
- 2½ C flour

Mix all ingredients, except flour, together well, then using your hands, work in the flour. Divide dough in three parts. Into one part, mix 1 oz. chocolate, in the other part a few drops red food coloring, mixing until dough is pale shade of pink. Leave other part as is. Force dough through cookie press on ungreased cookie sheet. Use different shapes. Mix some of the three shades of sough together for interesting effects. Bake 400 degrees 7-10 minutes.

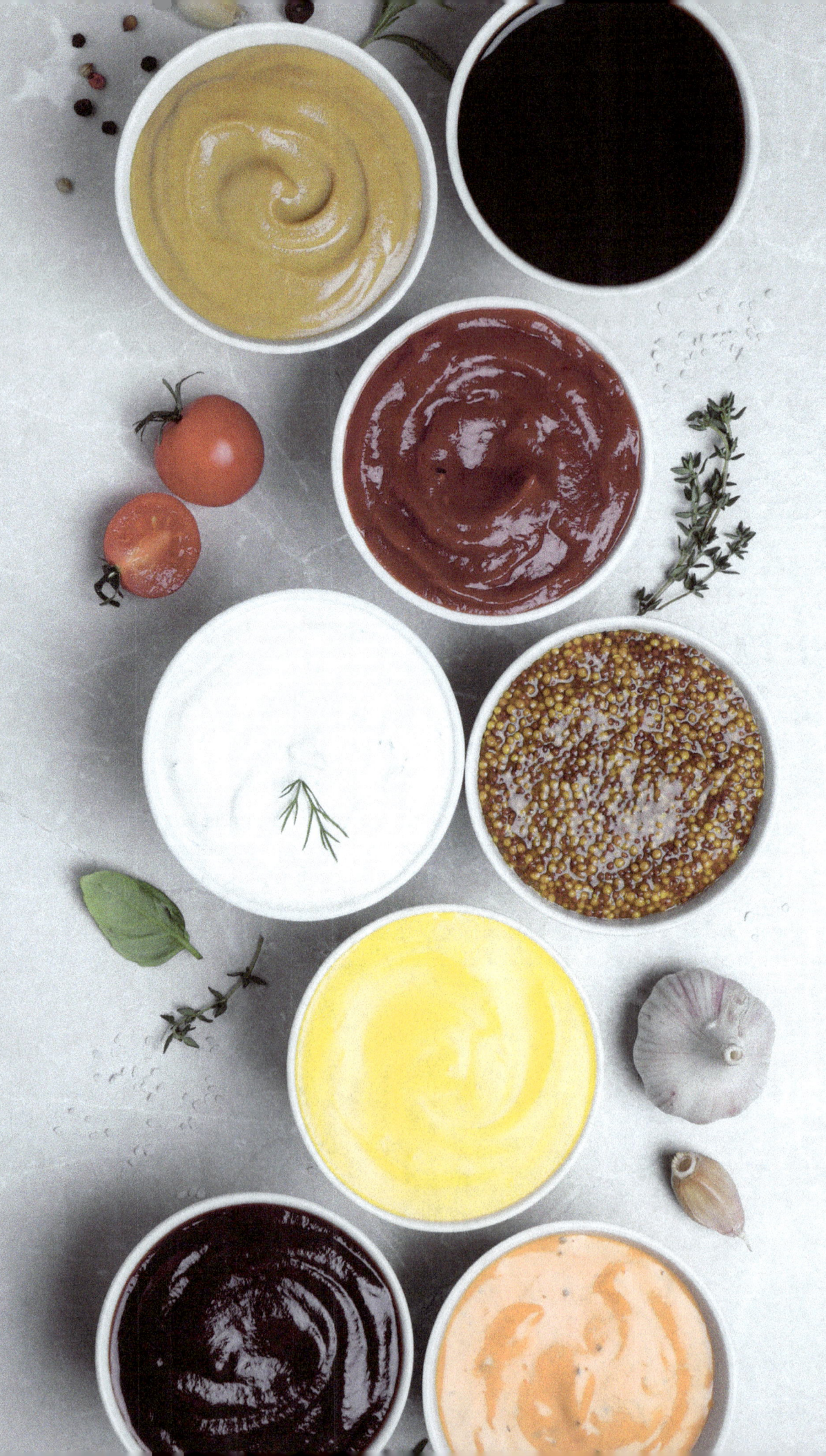

Frostings, Fillings & Sauces

Perhaps this is "Gilding the Lily" but there are times when some foods need 'gilding'...

A layer cake, without frosting, is just not a layer cake.

Where would spaghetti be without spaghetti sauce, etc.?

There are so many frostings, it was difficult to choose but I tried to include my favorites.

There are other toppings and fillings elsewhere in the book, they go with specific cakes but be creative; frost it, fill it and sauce it.

FRUIT DRESSING

- 1 C mayonnaise
- 1 3 oz. pkg. cream cheese, softened
- 2 T sugar
- About ¼ - ⅓ C fruit juice

Beat mayonnaise, cheese and sugar until well blended. Add fruit juice, a small amount at a time until the consistency of heavy cream.

THOUSAND ISLAND DRESSING

- 2 C mayonnaise
- ⅓ C ketchup or chili sauce
- ¼ C minced green onion
- 2 T pickle relish

Refrigerate for at least 1 hour before serving.

DELUXE VANILLA FROSTING

- 1 package vanilla frosting
- ¼ C finely chopped pecans
- ¼ C chopped maraschino cherries, well drained

Beat frosting according to directions. Add fruit and nuts. Delicious on a spice cake or rich yellow cake.

CHOCOLATE BUTTER FROSTING

- 2 C confectioner's sugar
- 1 egg
- ⅓ C soft butter or margarine
- 2 squares of unsweetened chocolate, melted
- ½ t vanilla

Beat at high speed until fluffy and right consistency for spreading.

DELUXE VANILLA FROSTING

- 1 package vanilla frosting
- ¼ C finely chopped pecans
- ¼ C chopped maraschino cherries, well drained

Beat frosting according to directions. Add fruit and nuts. Delicious on a spice cake or rich yellow cake. If frosting is too thin, add a few tablespoonful of confectioner's sugar.

VARIATIONS:

1. Add 2 T instant coffee
2. Add ½ C miniature marshmallows and ½ C chopped nuts
3. Add 2 T maraschino cherry juice and ½ C chopped cherries. Eliminate vanilla.

CHOCOLATE ORANGE FROSTING

- 1 package chocolate fudge frosting
- 1 T grated orange rind
- 2-3 T thawed concentrated orange juice

Beat on high speed until it reaches consistency for spreading. Enough for 2 layers or 13X9 inch cake.

CREAMY LEMON FROSTING

- 1 3 oz. package cream cheese
- 1 T lemon juice
- grated rind of one lemon
- 1½ C confectioner's sugar

Blend cheese, juice and rind; add sugar gradually until it reaches right consistency for spreading. Frosts one 8X8 cake.

GRASSHOPPER FILLING

- 1 envelope gelatin
- ¼ C cold water
- ⅓ C white creme de cocoa
- ⅓ C green creme de menthe
- 2 C whipped cream

Soften gelatin in cold water. Heat the liquors, stir in gelatin until dissolved; cool. Fold into whipped cream.

SOFT CUSTARD SAUCE

- 1 egg plus 1 yolk
- ¼ C sugar
- dash of salt
- 2 C scalded milk
- 1 t vanilla

Cook and stir over very low heat, until custard coats a spoon. Chill. Add about 1 t vanilla. Serve over plain cake or puddings.

MEDIUM WHITE SAUCE

- 3 T butter
- 3 T flour
- ¼ t salt
- dash of pepper
- 1 C milk

Melt butter, blend in flour, cook over low heat, stirring constantly until mixture bubbles. Remove from heat and slowly stir in milk. Bring to boil, stirring constantly, and boil 1 minute.

VARIATIONS:

Cheese sauce: add ½ C grated cheese, American, cheddar or Jack. Stir until cheese melts.

Egg and Olive sauce: add 2 hard cooked eggs, chopped and ¼ C black or green olives, chopped

HORSERADISH SAUCE

- ⅓ C prepared horseradish
- 1 C sour cream
- dash of sugar
- salt to taste

Mix together well. Serve cold with cold cuts.

MUSTARD SAUCE

- 2-3 T prepared mustard
- 1 C sour cream
- salt to taste

Mix until well blended. Serve with cold ham or pork.

EASY SPAGHETTI SAUCE

- 1 lb. 12 oz. can tomatoes
- 2 T oil
- 1 medium onion, sliced
- 1 clove garlic, minced
- 6 oz. can tomato paste
- ½ t Italian mixed spices
- ¼ t sugar
- salt to taste

Drain tomatoes and save liquid. Chop tomatoes and add to liquid. Lightly brown onion and garlic in oil, stir in tomatoes, tomato paste, spices, sugar and salt. Cover and boil gently 15 minutes then uncover and simmer for about 30 minutes until it thickens.

BLUEBERRY SAUCE

- ½ C sugar
- 1 ½ T corn starch
- 1 pt. blueberries
- ¾ C water
- 1 t lemon juice
- 1 T margarine

Blend sugar with corn starch, add berries, water and lemon juice. Cook, stirring constantly, until thickened and clear. Simmer for about 1 minute then stir in margarine. Cool slightly before serving.

PLUM SAUCE

- ½ C plum jam
- 1 ½ T wine vinegar
- 2 T soy sauce
- ½ t dry mustard

Boil 2 minutes, stirring constantly. Serve with Chinese food.

HAM GLAZE

- 1 t dry mustard or 2 T prepared mustard
- ¼ t cloves
- ½ C brown sugar
- 10 oz. can apricot or pineapple juice

Mix all ingredients together and pour over 5 lb. ham. Bake 1 hour in 350 degrees, basting often.

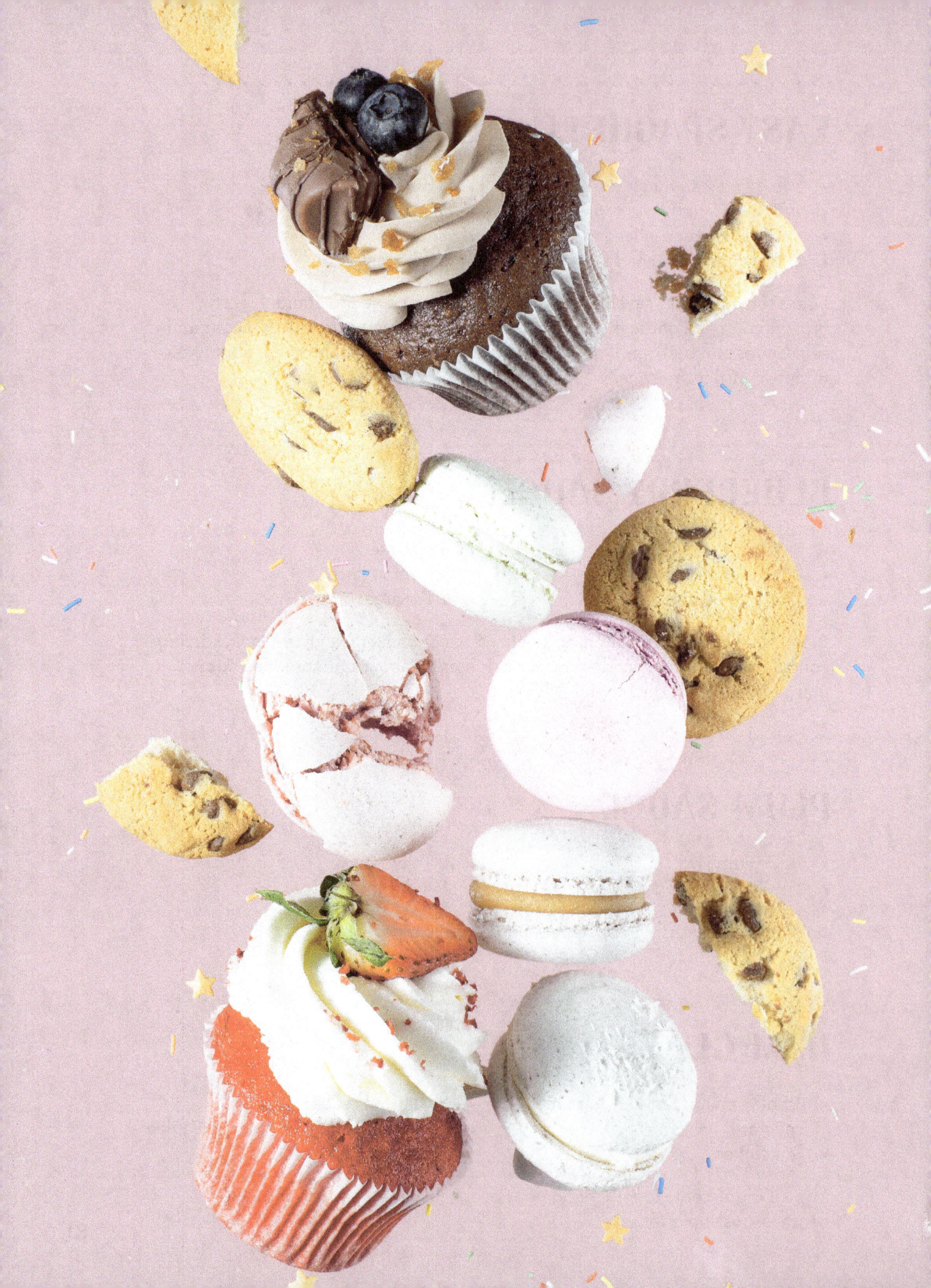

Desserts

The "Piece de Resistance".

To most of us the dessert brings the lament "I shouldn't really", but we go right ahead and partake.

Desserts vary from the cheese and fruit tray to the very rich pastries, heaped high with whipped cream and untold calories.

When serving a heavy meal, a light dessert would be in order. Fruit cup, sherbet or a gelatin would be a pleasant ending.

When a lighter meal or snack is served, a richer dessert may be served.

Pies and cakes are listed separately in this book.

FRUIT SALAD, Version 1

- 1 C cantaloupe balls
- 1 C honeydew melon balls
- 1 C watermelon balls
- 1 C fresh blueberries

Use all the juices that gather when cutting melons. If more juice is desired, pour ginger ale over fruit a few minutes before serving. Serve very cold.

FRUIT SALAD, Version 2

- 2 grapefruit
- 2-3 large naval oranges
- 1 C pineapple, fresh or canned
- 1 C peaches, fresh or canned
- 1 C strawberries, cut
- 1 tart apple, peeled and sliced
- ½ C orange juice
- ¼ C grenadine syrup or maraschino juice
- cherries or green seedless grapes

Cut grapefruit and oranges into segments, remove pits and membrane. Use all the juice. Add the rest of the fruit and juices. Serve very cold.

BREAD PUDDING

- 3 C milk
- 3 c bread cubes
- ¼ C melted butter
- ½ C sugar
- 3 eggs, slightly beaten
- 1 C chopped apples
- 1 t cinnamon
- ½ C raisins, (optional)

Heat milk to scalding and pour over bread cubes. When cool, add rest of the ingredients. Pour into 2 qt. casserole and bake 40-45 minutes 350 degrees.

GRAPENUT LEMON PUDDING

- ¾ C butter
- ½ C sugar
- 1 t grated lemon rind
- 2 egg yolks
- 3 T lemon juice
- 2 T flour
- ¼ C Grape-nuts
- 1 C flour
- 2 egg whites, slightly beaten

Cream butter, sugar, rind well. Add yolks, beat until fluffy. Blend in juice, cereal, milk (mixture will look curdled). Fold in egg whites. Pour in greased custard cups or 1 qt. casserole. Place in pan of hot water. Bake 325 degrees about 40 minutes or until top springs back when lightly touched.

FRUIT FRITTERS

- 1 C flour
- 2 t baking powder
- ¼ C sugar
- 1 t vanilla
- ¼ t cinnamon
- 1 egg, beaten
- ⅓ C milk
- 8 canned pineapple slices
- 8 canned peach halves, drained
- 8 canned pear halves, drained
- 2 solid bananas, cut in halves

Add liquids to dry ingredients. Mix well to a smooth batter. Dip well drained fruit in batter and deep fry until golden brown. Remove from oil and drain on paper towels.

Serve hot with powdered sugar.

CORN FLAKE PUDDING

- 5 C corn flakes
- 1 C chopped apples
- ½ C jam (raspberry, plum or strawberry)
- cinnamon
- sugar
- milk

Place layer of corn flakes in 1½ qt. baking dish. Cover with layer of apples, some jam, sugar and cinnamon. Repeat layers until dish is very full. Pour milk until it reaches ¾ of baking dish. Cover and bake 25-30 minutes in 350 degrees. Serve warm with light cream. Serves 4-6.

RICE PUDDING

- ½ C water
- ½ C instant rice
- 3 eggs, slightly beaten
- ½ C sugar
- 2 t vanilla
- ¼ t salt
- 2½ C scalded milk

Prepare rice as directed on box. Mix all ingredients together, sprinkle with cinnamon. Bake in ungreased casserole which has been placed in a pan of hot water. Bake 70 minutes at 350 degrees.

APPLE CRISP

- 6 apples
- ½ C margarine
- 1 t cinnamon
- ½ C brown sugar
- ½ C white sugar
- ½ C flour
- ½ C cold water

Slice apples. Blend all ingredients except water. Top apples with the crumbs. Add water. Cover and bake 350 degrees 1 hour. Fresh plums may be used instead of apples. Use about 2-1/2 lbs. fresh prune-plums and bake for 45 minutes.

FRUITED RICE

- 3 C cooked rice
- ½ C sour cream
- 2–3 T sugar
- ½ C miniature marshmallows
- ½ C drained chunk pineapple
- ¼ C mandarin oranges
- about 10 black or maraschino cherries, cut in halves

Mix together until well blended. Chill several hours. Serve with whipped cream as a dessert.

APPLE NOODLE PUDDING

- 8 oz. wide noodles
- 1 C chopped apples
- ¼ C chopped walnuts
- 3 eggs, beaten
- 1½ C sour cream
- ¼ t cinnamon
- 2½ T sugar
- ¼ C raisins (optional)

Cook noodles and drain. Add apples and nuts. Blend eggs, sugar, sour cream and cinnamon; Add to noodle mixture.

Melt butter in 1½ qt. casserole and pour in mixture. Bake 350 degrees 30-35 minutes or until top and sides are a golden brown. Serve with fruit sauce.

Miscellaneous

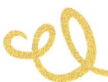 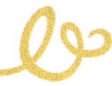

The heading "miscellaneous" can mean many things, but believe me it was not an afterthought to include "odds and ends".

These recipes are some of our very favorites, some have an ethnic background, others just don't come under any special classification.

Try them and perhaps you will add a new dish to your recipe file.

MOCK BLINTZES

- 1½ C cottage cheese
- 1 egg, slightly beaten
- 1 t cinnamon
- 2 T sugar
- 1 box Uneeda Biscuits
- 1 egg, beaten
- 1 T milk

Mix first four ingredients (left column above) together well and set aside. Mix milk and egg; dip crackers in egg mixture. Place about 1 tablespoon of cheese mixture on cracker and cover with another cracker. Dip each sandwich in egg mixture and fry in butter or margarine until golden brown. Serve plain or with cinnamon and sugar mixture.

BLINTZES (COTTAGE CHEESE)

BATTER
- 4 eggs, well beaten
- 1 C flour
- 1 t salt
- 1 C milk

FILLING
- 1½ lb. cottage cheese
- 2 yolks, beaten
- 2 T sugar
- 1 t cinnamon

For filling, mix all ingredients together. For batter, add liquid to salt and eggs, stirring in the flour gradually until smooth. Use a 6 inch skillet, greased with vegetable shortening. Pour a small amount of batter in skillet tipping from side to side to cover bottom. Bake on one side only. Turn out on clean towel, baked side up. When several pancakes have been made, place 1 T of filling in the center of each pancake, fold the side towards you over filling, then fold both sides towards center, then roll. Continue until batter and filling is used. Before serving, fry on both sides until golden brown. Serve hot with jam or sugar and cinnamon and sour cream. Also delicious with sliced and sugared strawberries.

KASHA (BUCKWHEAT GROATS)

- 1½ C medium kasha
- 1 egg
- ½ t salt

Mix together well set aside to dry. When dry mix with fork until the kasha is separated and there are no lumps. Place in 1½ qt. sauce pan and place pan over low heat, stirring constantly so as not to burn. When heated through, pour about 2¾ C boiling water over the hot kasha, do not let the boiling stop. Cover, lower flame, and cook until all water is absorbed and kasha is soft and each grain is separated. May be served as a side dish with pot roast; pour gravy over kasha, or brown 1 large onion and add to kasha, or cook 1 C pasta bows in salted water and add to onions then add to kasha.

MATZOTH PUDDING

- 2 Matzoth
- 2 eggs, well beaten
- 1 jar apple & pineapple, chunk style
- 1 T sugar
- ½ t cinnamon

Dampen matzoth and crumble. Add the rest of the ingredients. Bake in greased 2 qt. casserole about 35-40 minutes 375 degrees or until golden brown around edges.

MATZOTH BALLS

- 2 T chicken fat
- 2 eggs slightly beaten
- ½ C matzoth meal
- 1 t salt
- 2 T water

Mix fat and eggs together, add meal, salt and water. Cover, set in refrigerator for 1 hour or more. Make small balls and drop into salted boiling water. Cover and lower flame. cook for 30 minutes or until all balls float on top of water. Lift with slotted spoon. Add to chicken soup or serve as side dish with potato roast; pouring gravy over matzoth balls.

BREAD STUFFING

- 3½ dry bread cubes
- ½ onion, chopped
- ¼ C celery, chopped
- 1 egg
- 1 bouillon cube, dissolved in ½ C water
- salt and pepper

Combine ingredients. Mix well

STUFFING

- 4 C dried bread cubes
- ½ C melted shortening (chicken fat, extra good)
- 1 small onion, chopped
- ½ C celery, chopped
- chicken giblets, cooked and chopped
- salt, pepper, dash of poultry seasoning
- 1 egg, beaten plus 2 T water

Cook onion and celery until tender. Add giblets and shortening. Mix with bread cubes, add egg mixture. Stuff chicken or turkey lightly. If there is any stuffing remaining, bake it in a greased baking dish along with the fowl. Cut in squares and serve instead of potatoes.

PLANTAINS (MEXICAN BANANAS)

- 3 ripe plantains
- oil

Plantains should be very ripe, soft to the touch but not black. Peel and slice in ¼ inch slices. Fry in oil until golden brown on both sides. Serve as side dish to Mexican or Spanish food or with scramble eggs.

GARLIC BREAD

- 1 long loaf French or Italian bread, split lengthwise
- 1 t garlic powder or 2 cloves fresh garlic, crushed
- 1½ sticks of butter or margarine
- Parmesan cheese
- paprika

Soften butter or margarine, add garlic. Spread on both halves of bread, sprinkle generously with cheese and paprika. Wrap in aluminum foil and heat for about 10 minutes, then open folds of foil and heat for a few minutes more until brown and crisp.

www.ingramcontent.com/pod-product-compliance
Lightning Source LLC
Chambersburg PA
CBHW060426010526
44118CB00017B/2379